INSTANT LOSS
cookbook

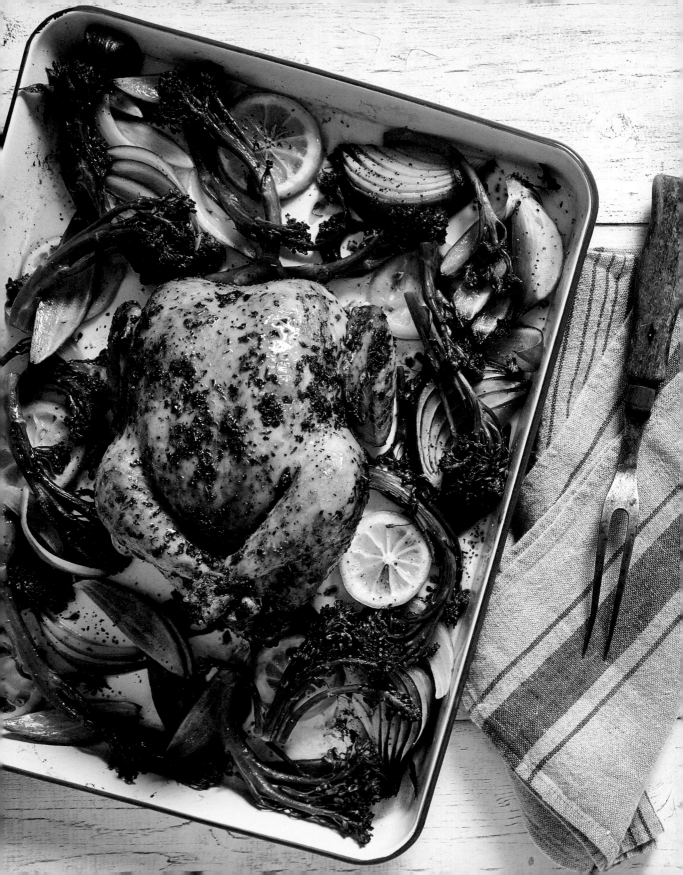

INSTANT LOSS
cookbook

Cook Your Way to a Healthy Weight with
125 Recipes for Your Instant Pot®,
Pressure Cooker, and More

Brittany Williams

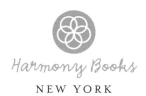

Harmony Books

NEW YORK

Copyright © 2018 by Brittany Williams

All rights reserved.
Published in the United States by Harmony Books,
an imprint of the Crown Publishing Group,
a division of Penguin Random House LLC, New York.
crownpublishing.com

Harmony Books is a registered trademark, and the Circle colophon
is a trademark of Penguin Random House LLC.

Some recipes originally appeared on the author's blog, https://instantloss.com.

Library of Congress Cataloging-in-Publication Data
Names: Williams, Brittany, 1989– author.
Title: Instant loss cookbook : cook your way to a healthy weight /
with 125 recipes for your instant pot, pressure cooker,
and more / [Brittany Williams].
Description: New York : Harmony Books, 2018. | Includes index.
Identifiers: LCCN 2018012570 (print) | LCCN 2018016646 (ebook) |
ISBN 9780525577249 (ebook) | ISBN 9780525577232 (trade pbk.)
Subjects: LCSH: Weight loss. | Pressure cooking. | Electric cooking, Slow. |
Quick and easy cooking. | LCGFT: Cookbooks.
Classification: LCC RM222.2 (ebook) | LCC RM222.2 .W45457 2018 (print) |
DDC 641.5/884—dc23
LC record available at https://lccn.loc.gov/2018012570

ISBN 978-0-525-57723-2
Ebook ISBN 978-0-525-57724-9

Printed in the United States of America

Book design by Ashley Tucker
Photographs by Hélène Dujardin
Cover design by Ashley Tucker
Cover photographs by Hélène Dujardin

10 9 8 7 6 5 4

First Edition

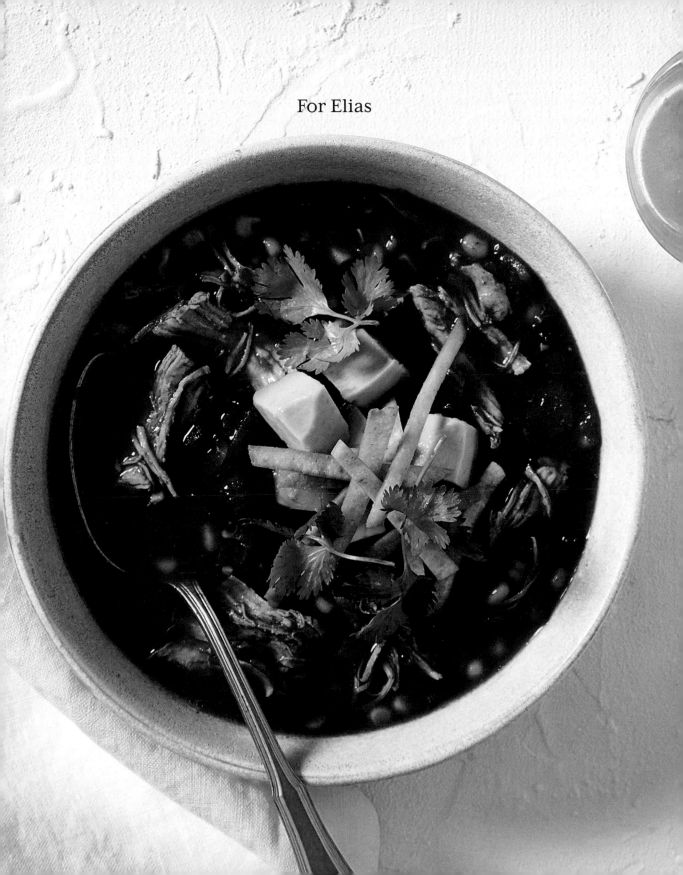

For Elias

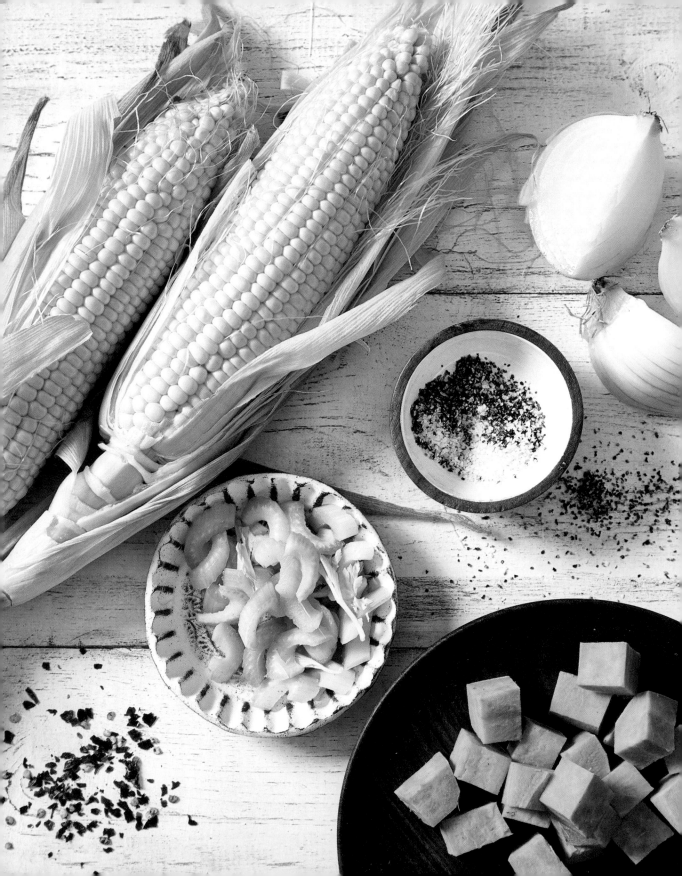

CONTENTS

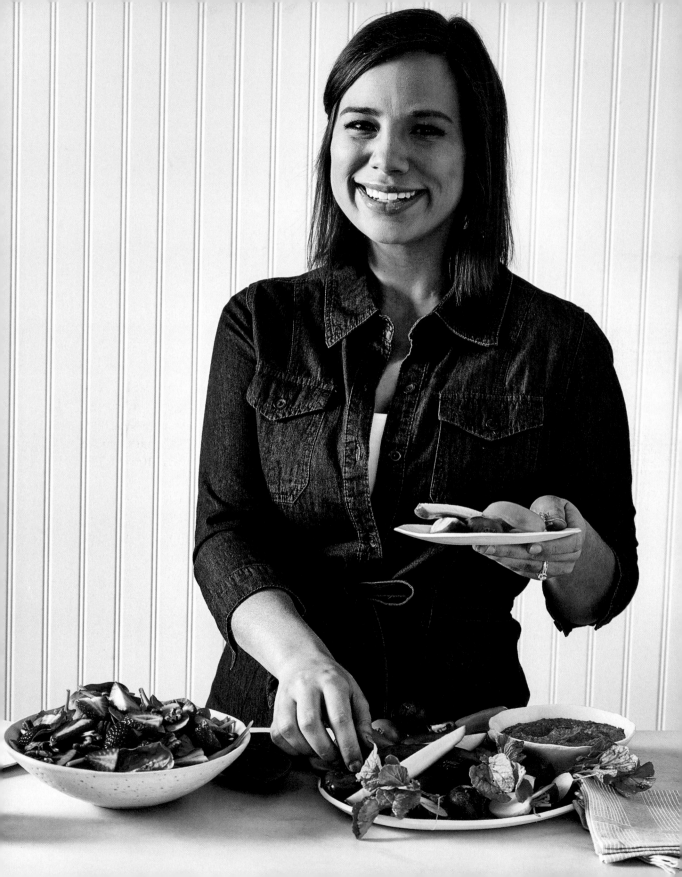

INTRODUCTION

December 2016

I remember December 2016 so clearly. The holiday parties had finally ended, and my countertops were littered with all sorts of sugary snacks: leftover Christmas cookies, pecan pies, red-and-white striped candy canes—even the air in my house smelled like delicious sugar confections. I was leaning against the counter, scrolling through Instagram, mindlessly nibbling on a piece of my Aunt Kim's famous homemade fudge.

With January right around the corner, I could feel it in the pit of my stomach: this year had to be different. The fact that I had never kept a single New Year's resolution didn't matter. There was going to be something special about 2017.

I knew I needed to make a change. I wanted to be healthy, but I didn't want to sacrifice flavor or eating foods I loved. Could I lose weight without diet pills, weight-loss schemes, multilevel marketing propaganda, surgery, or intense workout regimes? At my highest weight, I was 260 pounds. At 5'2¾" that's a lot to carry. Was it possible to lose 100 pounds naturally?

Almost everyone in my life who has lost large amounts of weight underwent gastric bypass surgery. It was something I'd considered, but I'd seen both ends of the spectrum: extreme success and horrible relapse. I knew that making my stomach smaller wasn't the solution.

This journey, for me, was going to be a mental battle.

My Story

This cookbook is a little different from most other cookbooks. It's like a cookbook plus a girlfriend who likes to talk.

You didn't know this was a two-for-one deal!

This is a collection of the 125 recipes plus meal plans that I used over the course of the year that I lost 125 pounds. These recipes are gluten free, dairy optional, pretty low in sugar, and high in healthy whole ingredients. There are lots of veggies, but you can also eat a cookie now and then. These are the recipes that support a healthy lifestyle—not a diet.

I also share personal information in this introduction because I want you to understand that this journey was a process. I've learned a lot about health and wellness during the last seven years, but between having babies, experiencing grief, and juggling a busy life, I lost weight just to gain it back . . . several times.

What made this time any different?

Like so many of us, I didn't grow up in a particularly healthy household. I grew up in Southern California, then moved to Texas at sixteen, in the days before Instant Pots, Gluten-Free, Whole 30, and Keto Diets were a thing. No one was talking about celiac, autoimmune protocols, or Paleo. When I was nine, my father suddenly became disabled after an accident and my mother began working overtime to support our family of nine. (Yes, you read that right. I'm the oldest of seven children.) Needless to say, healthy eating wasn't high on the priority list. We had our own version of important food groups: *fast*, *frozen*, *fried*, and *processed*. We lived on french fries, hot dogs, white bread, and sugar-filled cereal—things that we could make ourselves or could easily be procured with a trip to McDonalds. By the time I was a preteen, I was classified as overweight. At eighteen, I was already over 200 pounds.

Weight loss was central during my childhood. My parents were yo-yo dieters, always trying the next fad-thing to lose weight. There was SlimFast, the Hollywood Juice Diet, HCG, Lean Cuisines, Metabolife—you name it, my parents tried it. Countless times I watched them lose large amounts of weight only to gain it all back. That was my introduction to extreme and unhealthy dieting.

When I was sixteen years old I was diagnosed with an autoimmune disor-

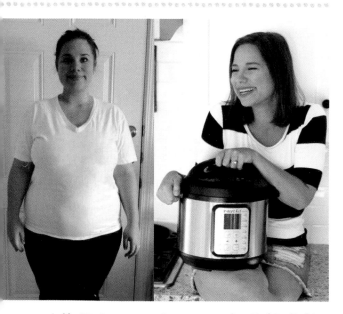

Left: Me in 2016, at 240 pounds. Right: Eight months later after losing 105 pounds.

der: hypothyroid disease. My mom found it peculiar that even though my eating patterns hadn't changed, I was packing on weight. My hair was also falling out in handfuls and I was dealing with insomnia and extreme fatigue. My doctor put me on Synthroid and told me that I would be on medication for the rest of my life. She told me that weight would always be a struggle because of my disease. Instead of being totally depressed about it, I felt as though someone gave me a magic "get out of jail free" card. Being overweight wasn't my fault. I could blame it on my disease!

This struggle with obesity continued into my adult life. I formed unhealthy attachments with food. If something great happened, I would reward myself with food. If something traumatic happened, I'd console myself with food. If I was on my period, if I was tired, if I was bored, if I was lonely, sad, happy, mad . . . one simple answer: *food*.

In the moment, food really did make me feel better.

But there's always the day after a binge. And I'd beat myself up over not having more control.

I began crash-dieting. I'd starve myself or resolve to eat only grilled chicken and broccoli. I'd stick to a juice diet for a while or count calories, and when that didn't work I counted points. But then life would get crazy and I wouldn't have time to track, so I invested in processed weight-loss meals, then gym memberships and personal trainers. I bribed myself with the promise of shopping sprees and vacations. I tried everything.

Nothing. Ever. Worked.

I started and stopped so many different diets that I lost count. My *entire* life revolved around the fact that I was fat and trying to get UNFAT so I could finally appreciate the girl on the outside as much as I liked the one on the inside.

I loved my inner self. Honestly, I thought I was a catch—on the inside. And I hated that I had to make that disclaimer. I just wanted to be an awesome catch. PERIOD.

I was SICK of never having clothes that fit me. Sick of going to the store and trying on the largest size, just to have it not fit either. Sick of breaking a sweat just trying to get pants on. Sick of breathing heavy and feeling winded after walking up a flight of stairs. Sick of being accused of being immodest because of my enormous chest size that, let me be frank, would have given me cleavage in a turtleneck.

I was TIRED of having to crop every photo of myself at the bust. I was TIRED of turning down invitations to go places because I was afraid of what old friends would think and say if they saw me so heavy. And I was REALLY TIRED of being too embarrassed to run around with my kids because of all the parts I had that jiggled.

I couldn't seem to shake myself out of it. I couldn't seem to climb out of the pit. I didn't know how to save myself. I didn't know how to break the cycle and reclaim my life.

. . . .

My husband, Brady, has always been con-cious of nutrition. He grew up the com-plete opposite of me—in every way, not just nutritionally. After we got married, I still remember the look of horror he gave me when I stuck a 97 cent loaf of white bread in our cart on our first trip to the grocery store together.

"Oh, Babe, we don't eat that! It's bleached, starved of nutrients, full of sugar, and preservatives!"

I looked at him funny. "I don't know what all those things are, but this is bread and bread is good."

I didn't have a clue. I had never heard of processed food, didn't know what GMO, MSG, aspartame, this dye, that dye was or any of the other bazillion ingredi-ents that we were apparently supposed to stay away from.

Brady is awesome, though. He kindly began to explain the ins and outs of ingredients to me. What they meant and why it's important. We started watching food documentaries together, like *Fat, Sick and Nearly Dead*, *Forks over Knives*, *GMO OMG*, and *Food Matters*, and I started to understand.

This whole time I'd been overcom-plicating food. If I just ate real food and invested in things like non-GMO, organic, pasture-raised, grass-fed ingredients instead of all the different "lose weight quick" schemes I had been investing in . . . well, I would be on to something.

There was a five-year period after we got married when I lost and regained a lot of weight. During this period we were having our children. I was 260 pounds after I had my first baby, Avey. In eighteen months, I lost 70 pounds then I got preg-nant with baby #2, Benjamin. I popped back up to 240 pounds after I had Ben-jamin. In another eighteen months I lost another 70 pounds, which put me in the 170s! I felt AMAZING. I promised myself that I'd never get heavy again.

But life doesn't ever seem to go as planned.

March 2015

Snow fell from the heavens all night long. In all my years of living in Texas, I had never seen so much snow. Thick, gor-geous layers of white covered our little home like a beautiful woolen blanket.

I was just a few days shy of being thirty-nine weeks pregnant with our third child, and I was eagerly awaiting the arrival of our midwife. I had suffered a miscarriage earlier that year, so being so close to the end was a relief. We couldn't wait to welcome our second son.

Brady was fixing a leak in the laun-dry room when our midwife arrived. She brought me flowers and we laughed and chatted about trivial things as I proudly gave her a tour of our little home.

We sat barefoot on the floor, our snow-covered boots at the door as I filled out paperwork and our son's birth certifi-cate. "Any day now . . ." we kept saying. He was our third full-term baby and I didn't expect to be pregnant much longer.

We relocated to the bedroom and my kids piled around as our midwife used her fetal Doppler to check on baby #3. My daughter, Avey, always the helper, took a turn with the Doppler. I noticed that it was taking longer than normal to find his heartbeat. "He must be in a strange position," I thought.

Minutes passed and my midwife put her Doppler away and smiled at me, her eyes bright and glassy like she was holding in tears. "It's time to go," she whispered.

"Go where?" I whispered back.

"To the hospital."

"Okay."

I don't know why, but I didn't ask her any questions. Maybe my spirit already knew the answers. Brady and I drove hand in hand to the hospital, navigating the snowy roads. He didn't say much but I talked the whole way.

"I know he's fine. Her Doppler must not be working. He's just in a funny position. I just felt him moving." I was trying to convince myself as much as I was trying to convince Brady.

After filling out some paperwork, they ushered me into a room where the ultrasound tech came in and set up without saying a word. We held our breath.

The room was still.

We knew right away.

I had never seen my husband cry before. All I could think was "take me back to this morning," sitting at the dining room window, filling out his birth certificate. Let me have just one more moment before my whole world crumbles.

I delivered him quietly. I only got to hold him for a few minutes before they carried him away. He was perfect. Looked just like his sister. Had the longest little fingers and toes you've ever seen.

The months after we lost Elias were the hardest months of my life. To add to the pain, we miscarried our next baby as well. I was in a fog that I now know was depression. I pushed people away like I did my emotions. I wanted to be numb. It was easier to operate from that space, rather than deal with my feelings.

For the first time, my "go-to fix-it" food didn't make me feel better. Nothing could make me feel better.

And yet, there was collateral beauty all around me: the women who cleaned my house and took care of my children while I recovered, the meals that were brought to me, the prayers that were said, the strangers online who raised money to pay for Elias's funeral and our medical bills. I felt so many things, but I *never* felt alone.

From a physical health perspective, gaining tremendous amounts of weight during pregnancy, just to end up with empty arms was difficult to reconcile. After I delivered my first two children, I started trying to lose weight immediately. But after Elias, none of that seemed important anymore. It took a life-changing diagnosis in the family to bring me back to myself.

A Life-Changing Diagnosis

I'll never forget the sheer panic that struck my heart when I was awakened to the pained cries of my four-year-old daughter, Avey, on February 10, 2016. She was screaming in agony, "Mommy! My whole body hurts! I can't get out of bed, I can't walk! Mommy, help!"

My husband raced up the stairs, taking them three at a time, and rushed her down to our bedroom. She had a fever of 106°F. Even more alarming was the way the joints in her fingers, toes, knees, elbows, and ankles literally ballooned before our eyes.

We called her pediatrician, who ordered us to the children's hospital ER without delay. And twenty-four hours later we had a diagnosis: juvenile polyarticular arthritis.

This was the worst case the Dallas Children's Hospital rheumatology team had ever seen in a child her age. Literally every joint in her little body had been affected. They immediately started her on a regimen of heavy-duty narcotics and NSAIDS (nonsteroidal anti-inflammatory drugs). As a relatively holistic mama, my kids had never even had Tylenol before. The thought of putting my four-year-old on weekly doses of medication used in chemotherapy treatment was terrifying.

I was desperate to find any alternative method of care. Having an autoimmune disease myself, hypothyroid disease, I knew there were special diets out there for the immuno-compromised designed to decrease inflammation in the body. I asked the rheumatology team if they had seen success in patients with diet change. I was told emphatically that diet change would not help, but to try it if it made me feel better.

I began researching and started to ask for all kinds of testing: leaky gut, food sensitivities, yeast overgrowth, parasites, gene mutations, and obscure testing for diseases that are known to trigger rheumatoid arthritis (RA). Her team of physicians told me that none of the testing I was asking for mattered. But I knew that our bodies weren't designed to attack themselves.

Feeling as though we had no other choice, and going against my better instincts, we decided to follow their treatment recommendations. This unfortunately made things so much worse. I saw my sweet little girl change. She became a different person. She was no longer the carefree, playful, fun little girl. Instead, she became angry and aggressive. She started saying crazy things, like she wished she was dead. Remember, she was four. She experienced terrible side effects from the medication. Desperate to get her off the supposedly helpful but unhelpful and harmful medication, I knew I had to find something else, some other course of treatment.

A Different Diet

My Dad was diagnosed with rheumatoid arthritis when he was in his forties and noticed that his symptoms would all but disappear when he took business trips to Southern California. After months of dealing with the torturous side effects of Avey's medications, I packed her up along with her two brothers, Benjamin and Noah, then three years old and two months, respectively, and headed to Southern California. Within two weeks of making this move, the change in our environment resulted in more of an improvement than we had seen in six months on medication.

By this time my husband and I had done countless hours of study on the effects of changes in barometric pressure and how it correlated with an increase of inflammation in the body. Because Texas has frequent pressure changes and high humidity, the weather was literally making her sick.

Additionally, even though our rheumatologist made it clear that she didn't believe diet change would make any difference with Avey's inflammation, we made the choice to try the Autoimmune Protocol (AIP) diet. This diet is a very strict diet and eliminates inflammatory, gut-irritating foods. This meant no grains, dairy, nightshades, legumes, or processed foods.

Thankfully, the change in climate coupled with the change in diet brought Avey into remission and she was able to go off *all* medication. After about six months, we began adding certain foods back into her diet that she seemed to tolerate well. Slowly, she began eating tomatoes, beans, corn, and gluten-free grains. Seeing her make such a miraculous recovery sparked something within me.

After Avey was diagnosed, we had cut a lot of foods out of our diet. Some nights there were tears about how unfair it was, but that didn't shake my resolve. During this time, I would eat with the kids during the day, but I would binge at night after they went to bed. I'd eat buckets of ice cream and send my husband to Sonic for double cheeseburgers, tots, and slushies.

I blamed it on stress and the fact that I was carrying a lot of heavy stuff.

As mothers we have an intense physical need to protect our children and keep them from harm; all born out of love in its deepest form. It doesn't matter if they get upset because we won't allow them to play in the street, as playing in the street is dangerous and it's our duty to protect them. In the same way, it doesn't matter if my kids really want junk food. I love them too much to allow them to poison their bodies. I love Avey too much to sit by and watch her make herself suffer. *Why couldn't I love myself that much?*

I was killing myself with food.

I had two choices. I could go on justifying my behavior or I could change. In 2016, I lost nearly fifty pounds by switching to a whole foods diet: vegetables, fruits, eggs, chicken, lean meat, herbs, nuts, seeds, and superfoods. I went from 260 pounds to 211 pounds.

But I quickly hit a plateau that I just couldn't break through. It was discouraging to eat so well and see zero progress. It was astonishing that at 5'2¾", and eating a largely plant-based diet, my body was retaining the weight it should have been shedding.

My Aunt Kim had been encouraging me for the last several years to get tested for a gene mutation that sounds more like a curse than anything else: MTHFR. Not knowing what else to do and completely out of new things to try, I got tested.

MTHFR stands for methylenetetrahydrofolate reductase gene. When functioning properly, it produces healthy MTHFR enzymes. When the gene is mutated, it creates an enzyme that is not correct.

It didn't come as a surprise to discover that I have two copies of the A1298C mutation. This means I inherited one from each of my parents. Because of this, I have 30 to 40 percent reduced enzyme functionality, have trouble methylating B vitamins, and have a complete intolerance for anything containing folic acid. Folic acid is essentially poison to my body.

Startlingly, this is not just the case for me but also for an estimated 40 to 60 percent of the population. If you've struggled with infertility, birth defects, miscarriage, or infant loss, **you need to be tested** for this mutation and begin supplementing accordingly.

The good news is that this mutation is very manageable with a diet rich in folate (while avoiding folic acid) and the proper methylated vitamins.

Within two weeks of being on the proper supplements, I broke through my weight-loss plateau and lost an astonishing ten pounds in one week. The next week I lost eight pounds! My hypothyroid disease went into remission, and I was able to go off my meds completely. It's like someone handed me the answer. My autoimmune disease was simply an outward indicator of my root sickness. The foods I had been eating my whole life were literally poisoning me. My autoimmune disease was a beacon for help from my body.

I cannot express enough the importance of finding and working with a functional medicine doctor if you have an autoimmune condition. Our bodies were not meant to destroy themselves. If you have an autoimmune condition, your body is trying to tell you something in the only way that it knows how. Please consult with your physician or a naturopath who is interested in digging into your disease and finding the underlying issue. This will change your life!

Enter Instant Pot

Brady is a gadget guy. He loves things that are electronic and come with the "supposed to make your life easier" label. One day he came home with an Instant Pot and a smile, sure that he was about to win the Husband of the Year award. I stared at that thing like it was my nemesis.

I don't really know why I felt so intimidated by it, but just gussying up the courage to take it out of the box took me *weeks*. I had small children and generally felt overwhelmed most of the time. The thought of trying to learn a whole new method of cooking gave me anxiety.

Before leaving for work one morning, my husband asked me if he should just return it. If he hadn't looked so sad about it I would have told him yes! By that point, it had sat in our living room for so long it had become part of the furniture. I didn't want to disappoint him, though, so instead I promised to try to use it that day for lunch.

I read the manual cover to cover. Still feeling confused about how I was supposed to use it, I decided to jump right in and make brown rice. And it was a smashing success! Not only was it crazy-delicious, but my kids ate the entire potful and I had to make more.

In January 2017, I issued myself a personal challenge: make dinner every night for an entire year. I was confident that with the help of my Instant Pot, I could achieve this.

I knew that in order to succeed, I needed something that made cooking easy and convenient. I had to quit eating out because I knew I didn't have the self-control or the willpower to say no. I was addicted to sugar and processed food.

Confident that I finally had all the tools I needed to be successful, I went through my cupboards, refrigerator, and freezer and threw out and gave away anything that would hinder progress.

If Avey couldn't eat it, I wouldn't eat it either (even in secret). It helped that we'd already been through the AIP diet and that I'd been cooking gluten free and (mostly) dairy free for my kiddos. Because of this, it wasn't a very drastic change.

There are nights I don't start cooking dinner till 6 p.m. because I lose track of time or we don't get home till late; there are nights that I used to pull out a frozen pizza or have my husband grab dinner on his way home from work. My Instant Pot has eliminated those nights. I can throw a few things in the pot and have dinner on the table in under a half hour.

I jumped in, all the way.

By February 2017, I had lost nineteen pounds. By the third month (March 2017), I was down forty-six pounds. As I continued to stay diligent in eating whole, nonprocessed foods, drinking enough water, and eating appropriate portions, the pounds continued to fall off. Then, in August 2017, I hit 135 pounds and decided to go into maintenance mode. I had lost 76 pounds in seven months, 125 pounds total!

When someone hears about another person losing weight, they usually want to know how they did it. The version of this question I most often received was: "What are you eating?" People wanted to know the specific details of my diet plan.

The J.E.R.F. Principal

My diet is simple: *Just eat real food* (J.E.R.F.). In our family, we restrict dairy, refined sugar, and gluten because we have auto-immune issues. Our issues don't respond well to those food groups, so we avoid them. Dairy, refined sugar, and gluten are also extremely inflammatory and most dietitians recommend at least limiting your consumption of grains, sugar, and dairy if you're trying to lose weight.

In conjunction with following the J.E.R.F. principal, I developed a different perspective of what food is meant to be: *fuel for my body*. And the way my body looks and feels is a reflection of the fuel I'm giving it. But while my mind wanted to fuel my body with natural, unprocessed ingredients, my taste buds felt differently. I knew I had to start gradually so I could stick to it.

This process started with limiting my grain consumption. Most days I do not eat grains at all. Twice a week, I'll have half a cup of organic brown rice or a couple homemade mini muffins that contain organic oats and are not fortified with folic acid.

I limit my dairy. I do eat a little bit of cheese here or there; some things are just too good to give up (like parmesan and cheddar!).

I do not eat sugar, with the exception of a little bit of raw local honey or grade A/B organic maple syrup. Sugar is what yeast needs to grow. Most Americans have leaky gut, which is a bacterial imbalance fueled by sugar. If you are eating processed, prepackaged, middle-of-the-grocery-store foods, you really can't avoid these things.

I eat loads of veggies. I try to "eat the rainbow" every day. Making sure my fruit and vegetables are various colors is a simple way to remember that eating a variety of fruits and vegetables will provide all the vitamins and nutrients you need. I do it up heavy on the green. Indeed, vegetables are the majority of what I eat at every meal.

I limit fruit because it has naturally occurring sugars that I don't want to eat too much of while I'm trying to lose weight. For example, I eat half an apple or half a banana and a handful of berries in a smoothie. That's about all the fruit I eat in a day. Lemons are an exception because they're so low in sugar.

I also eat eggs, meat, alternative flours (coconut, almond, and cassava), oils (coconut, avocado, and olive), nuts, seeds, and dark chocolate.

I drink at least ten 8-ounce glasses of water a day. The body needs water to release toxins and make the bowels move. Water also increases the rate at which you burn calories and can increase your metabolism by up to 70 percent!

At meals, I remind myself that my stomach is only as big as my fist, if I eat any more than that it can cause distention. Eating in this manner means that I tend to eat a little more frequently. I usually eat three meals a day with one to two snacks interspersed throughout the day.

The best thing about eating this way is that it's NOT a diet (as we typically view diets). It's exactly the way we all should be eating. I've been successful eating this way largely because I prepare all my own food. I can have the chocolate chip cookie I made myself with honey and almond flour instead of the store-bought, heavily processed, nutrient-starved cookie made from fortified wheat flour, and tons of sugar.

There are no secrets, there is no plan; it's just eating the right foods, in the right portions, and making sure I'm armed with the right tools, so that even on nights I don't feel like cooking, I don't call the pizza man.

We keep breakfast very simple in my house. If you start the day right, it's easier to stay on track. A fulfilling breakfast also prevents me from snacking between breakfast and lunch. My breakfasts usually consist of a green smoothie, eggs, and turkey bacon or a frittata. For lunch, I fill up on a big salad or a veggie tray with Homemade Ranch Dressing (page 98). After lunch, I'm always super-hungry around 2 or 3 p.m., because of this, I like to have a healthy snack at my fingertips, like hummus and veggies, apples and peanut butter, or hard-boiled eggs. Dinner is the meal that requires the most thought in our home. With a busy family of five, I like to cook things that don't take more than thirty minutes to prepare. Usually that means making something in my pressure cooker; a soup, stew, or quinoa bowl. Be diligent in preparing meals beforehand, as this is truly the key to success. Having ingredients, snacks, meal plans, leftovers, and frozen meals on hand sets you up for success.

When I was overweight, one of my biggest pitfalls was binge eating at night. It happened after dinner, after the kids were asleep, while Brady and I were catching up on TV. In order to change how I ate, I also had to make adjustments to my lifestyle. So, in cutting out processed, unhealthy food, we also cut out the triggers that were associated with it. We stopped watching TV. I had to replace how we relax at the end of the day. Now Brady and I play board games, we work on projects together, or we spend our time alone, being creative. Since these activities are more engaging than watching TV, I don't fall into the trap of eating mindlessly. So many unhealthy calories are consumed when you don't even realize it. When I say we made a lifestyle adjustment, I mean we not only adjusted what we ate but we also adjusted how, where, and why!

Why I Don't List Nutritional Information

There are several reason why I do not list nutritional information in this book or on my website. Mainly, it's because I spent years tracking calories, carbs, points, micros, and macros with little to no success. As soon as I stopped tracking, the weight began to creep back on—and who has time to count their food every day for the rest of their life?

I needed to retrain my mind to stop thinking about food as numbers and start thinking about it as fuel. I needed to stop obsessing over the numbers and start getting in touch with my body. I needed to understand the signals that it naturally sends about how it's being nourished and when I've had enough. For me, nutritionals were a stumbling block that had my mindset in "diet" mode instead of "this is just the way I eat" mode.

Another reason is that ingredients have different nutritional information. I can list the nutritionals based on the ingredients I use, but it would vary depending on the ingredients you're using. If you need to track nutritional information because you have a medical condition, it's best to calculate nutritional information yourself, with your own ingredients.

How to Start

Okay, so you bought this book either because you're trying to find inspiration for simple, yet yummy, healthy meals, or you're looking to shed unwanted weight. Either way, I'm so excited for you. Regardless of your motivation, if you cook from the *Instant Loss Cookbook* you will see and feel a difference, whether it's weight loss, increased energy, less bloating, or better sleep.

To set yourself up for success, here is a list of things to do:

1 **Take a "before" photo** and record your starting measurements and weight. Do not skip the measurements. There will be weeks where you may not lose any weight but you'll still lose inches. This can be a huge encouragement on your journey.

2 **Clean out your refrigerator and pantry.** Get rid of all heavily processed foods. To save on cost, things like condiments can stay around until you use them up. After they're consumed, purchase a healthier alternative. For example, use up your soy sauce and then replace it with coconut aminos. If you're really feeling motivated and want to clean out your entire pantry, consider donating any unopened goods to your local food pantry or shelter.

3 **Restock with whole foods.** That means lots of lean meats and veggies. And this is where the planning comes in. In this book, I've included one month of meal plans. You can mix and match as you see fit, but try not to put two carb-heavy meals together in one day. An easy formula to follow when you're starting to design your own meal plans is:

BREAKFAST = veggie-heavy smoothie or egg dish

LUNCH = salad with protein, leftovers, or something light on carbs (quinoa, brown rice, beans, oats are okay) and heavy on veggies. Check out anything from the soups, wraps, sides, vegetables, and salads sections.

DINNER = something family friendly and heavier on carbs is okay; just watch your portion sizes. For example, any of the one-bowl meals, kid food, or lunch/dinner options.

Lunch and dinner are interchangeable. Ideally, eat a carb-heavy meal at lunch.

4 **Focus on portion sizes.** Forget about counting calories, carbs, or points. Earlier in human history, diets were more plant based and less carb/meat based, and their portion sizes were much, much smaller. To emulate this, I use a small salad plate or a 1- or 2-cup bowl to measure my portions.

As a rule of thumb for portion size, I keep in mind that my stomach should ideally be the size of a clenched fist. Ideally the portion I eat shouldn't be much more than that. Eating more than a proper portion can cause my stomach to grow larger, which then causes me to need more food in the future to feel "full."

I try never to eat more than half a cup of quinoa or brown rice a day, I keep my meat protein at about 3 ounces per meal, and I fill my plate with as many vegetables as I like. If I go back for seconds, it's for the vegetable contents, not the heavy carbs or protein.

This also eliminates mindless eating. Sit at the table and think about the food as you're eating it. Think about how good it tastes and savor every bite. Set your fork or spoon down in between bites to give yourself more time to determine whether your body is beginning to feel full or not. Any leftovers are better in the fridge or even in the trash than in your body.

If you're still hungry after a meal, feel free to have a second helping of vegetables. Just do not take second helpings of heavy carbs: fried rice, quinoa bowls, or corn tortillas. Sometimes I just eat raw veggies with my avocado-veggie dip if I feel like I need a little something extra after a meal.

5 **The kitchen is closed after 7 p.m.** It's important to have a fasting period of time to allow your body to break down food and fat stores. If you're constantly eating, your body is constantly expending energy digesting your food. If you have a 12-hour+ time during the day when you abstain from eating, that energy is diverted to help break down fat stores.

6 **Get at least 8 hours of sleep every night.** Some of these steps are difficult depending on what stage of life you're in. I still have a one-year-old who shares our bed, and I haven't had eight hours of uninterrupted sleep in the last seven years, but that doesn't change the fact that getting enough sleep can greatly aid in weight loss and reducing stress.

7 **Track EVERYTHING.** I don't count points, micros, or calories, but I do keep track of what I'm eating, drinking, and what I weigh. I have a daily planner in which I write what I've eaten, how many ounces of water I've had, and what my weigh-in is for that day. This is an accountability tool that helps me stay on track and recognize patterns in my weight fluctuations and the food that I'm eating.

I do not advise that everyone weigh in every day. I know that this is a super touchy subject. The scale was a great accountability partner for me throughout my journey. It was a valuable tool to help me realize what foods my body liked to hold onto and what foods were easier to digest. I know that it's not such a positive thing for all of us, though, and I always recommend doing what is best for you and your mental health.

8 Drink, at the very least, eight 8-ounce glasses of water a day. I try to drink between ten and twelve glasses. Hydrating your body properly is key to losing weight, ridding your body of toxins, and cleaning out your bowels. I'm going to put this next part in capital letters: YOU MUST DRINK ENOUGH WATER IF YOU WANT TO BE SUCCESSFUL.

Carry water bottles with you wherever you go, buy a big old jug, do whatever it takes. Add citrus, fruit, or other natural flavors to the water if it is tough for you to drink. But whatever you do, make water your friend. This step is arguably the most important one.

9 Just MOVE. No need to get a fancy gym membership or spend hours on the treadmill, unless that's your thing, and then you ROCK! Like many of you, I work full time, I'm a mom of three, and I home-school my kids. I'm not making excuses, I'm just being realistic. My movement comes from chasing and playing with my kids. And when I do have a quiet moment, I want to sit down, not run to a gym.

I tried to do a YouTube "Yoga for Beginners" class once, and it was an utter disaster. My kids were climbing all over me. I kept having to restart the video, and my youngest kept trying to nurse anytime I got down on his level. The stage of life I'm in really isn't conducive to traditional workouts the way we typically think about working out.

So, let's start thinking about it differently! Do you sweep your floor or vacuum? That's exercise!

Scouring the bathroom totally counts! Taking a walk around the block and pulling your kids in a wagon; awesome arm workout! Babywearing while you cook, do chores, and fold laundry? Who needs an elliptical? Dancing with your babies while you do the dishes and prepare lunch, everyone wins!

Adding a few extra simple movements to your day will yield BIG results in the long run!

10 Dessert. Once a week, I'll make a treat for my family. I've always loved to bake. It helps me de-stress and my kids really love it. Friday night is our family dessert night. On this night, I usually make cookies, cake, or brownies, but I substitute traditional ingredients with healthier alternatives. Even though the treats have healthier ingredients, I still keep my portions in check.

Because I have healthier dessert substitutes at my fingertips, I don't feel that

I need to stuff my face and overindulge. I remind myself that I can make these kinds of treats again next week and still stay on track.

11 **Alcohol limits.** My husband and I had slipped into the unhealthy habit of drinking alcohol at night before bed. He'd have a beer and I'd have a glass of wine while watching Netflix and eating chips and salsa. In January, my goal wasn't to lose the weight as fast as I could. My goal was to make this lifestyle change sustainable for me, long term. And since alcohol was one thing that I really enjoyed, something had to give.

Instead of cutting out alcohol completely though, I decided to stop buying wine (mainly because there are no ingredients/nutritional facts listed) and start making my own skinny cocktails (see page 214). For the first month or two, I was still drinking an 8-ounce cocktail every other night. I was still able to lose weight, but surprisingly, my want for my nightcaps eventually waned and now I only drink socially, around once a month.

12 **Eat more frequently.** Because my portions are an appropriate size for me, I eat more frequently, usually three to six times a day. This typically consists of three meals with two to three small snacks interspersed. This keeps my metabolism up and prevents me from ever feeling "starved," which by default, keeps me from overindulging.

13 **Don't cook an award-worthy masterpiece meal six times a day.** I'm not cooking to win a James Beard Award. I'm cooking to fuel my and my family's bodies. I'm cooking to be healthy and I'm cooking to create the change in lifestyle. You'll find that my recipes use accessible ingredients and don't take too long to prepare or cook (I'm a mom of three kids!!), but boy, do they taste yummy. Just remember the whole trinity of meal time: *fat, fiber, protein.* Eating foods together that are rich in these three categories will help you burn more fat and stay fuller longer!

14 **Set yourself up for success! Get everyone on board.** Don't keep food that you don't want to eat inside your home—not for your husband, not for your kids, not for anyone. No exceptions. By keeping food like this around, you're setting yourself up for failure. If it's not around, you can't eat it.

I told everyone in my family what I was doing and why. I needed my family's help to keep me accountable until I was strong enough to do it on my own.

15 **Be kind to yourself.** We all make mistakes. We all have slip-ups, we're all trying our best. Don't beat yourself up. Be kind to yourself. Congratulate yourself that you're looking to make a positive change in your life. Recognize the road ahead might not be easy. You got this!

If I can do it,
you can do it!

Hour by hour, day by day, week by week, month by month—before you know, it's a way of life. It takes 21 days to form a healthy habit. I know you can do this for twenty-one days. I've included a thirty-day meal plan in this book. If you can get through three weeks of clean eating, you can make this a sustainable, long-term health change that will radically improve the quality of your life forever. Our bodies are the only things that are with us our entire lives, beginning when we begin and ending when we end. We have one chance to treat them right. Join me on this journey. You are worth it.

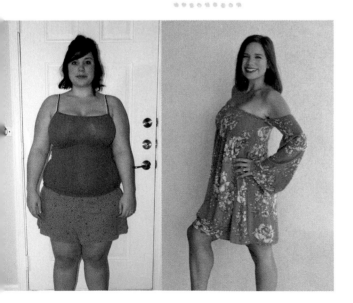

Reflecting on the Year: A Letter to Readers

My body tells my story. I'm a mama who carried six babies. I was unhealthy and now I am strong. I am richly and abundantly blessed to wear the skin that I have.

Reflection was an important part of my journey. Who am I doing this for? Who am I trying to please? If at any point the answer to those questions was anyone besides myself, I knew that it was time to stop.

My thighs still jiggle and touch. My body bares the markings of my story. And you know what? I am totally okay with that. Really, truly! My body has been through a lot and my appearance is a reflection of that. It doesn't upset me; it makes me proud. The weight wasn't the root of my problem, it was just an outward indicator that the inside of my body was sick.

This journey has been largely one of self-discovery and an exercise in self-control. It hasn't been easy, it hasn't been instant, but boy, has it been worth it. I'm a better wife, mother, and human being because of it. Not because I'm thinner now, but because I am more in tune with my body, mentally and physically. I am more disciplined with myself, I am more loving toward myself, and most important, I am more forgiving of myself.

I thought that I was setting out to lose weight, but I was really setting out to break the strongholds and addictions in my life concerning food. Every morning

I wake up, I have an opportunity to love myself better. I have an opportunity to look in the mirror and speak to the beautiful qualities within my spirit. To speak life over the body that blessed me with six beautiful pregnancies, to say thank-you for the arms that get to rock my earth babies and the legs that propel me forward. I have the blessed opportunity to be grateful for the chest that nourished three tiny humans and the face that my husband desperately loves. I have come to realize that my weight-loss struggle wasn't a struggle with weight at all. It was a heart struggle. Hearts need nourishment, too.

As you flip through the pages of this cookbook, you will find recipes to nourish your body, but I hope you will also be inspired to begin to take the time, if you haven't already, to invest in yourself by nourishing your soul. Let's get real. You're not going to drop 50 pounds overnight; this isn't some miracle cure. It takes hard work, perseverance, and time. But one thing I can assuredly promise you is that you will never regret investing in yourself.

This is your time, your year, your moment. There's nothing that I did that you can't do, too!

I'm writing this all curled up on my couch, wearing the ugliest wool socks you've ever seen and thinking about how to convey how grateful I am that you've allowed me to share my story with you. If you take nothing else away from this book, take this: *You're not alone.*

Wishing you success on your health journey,

Brittany

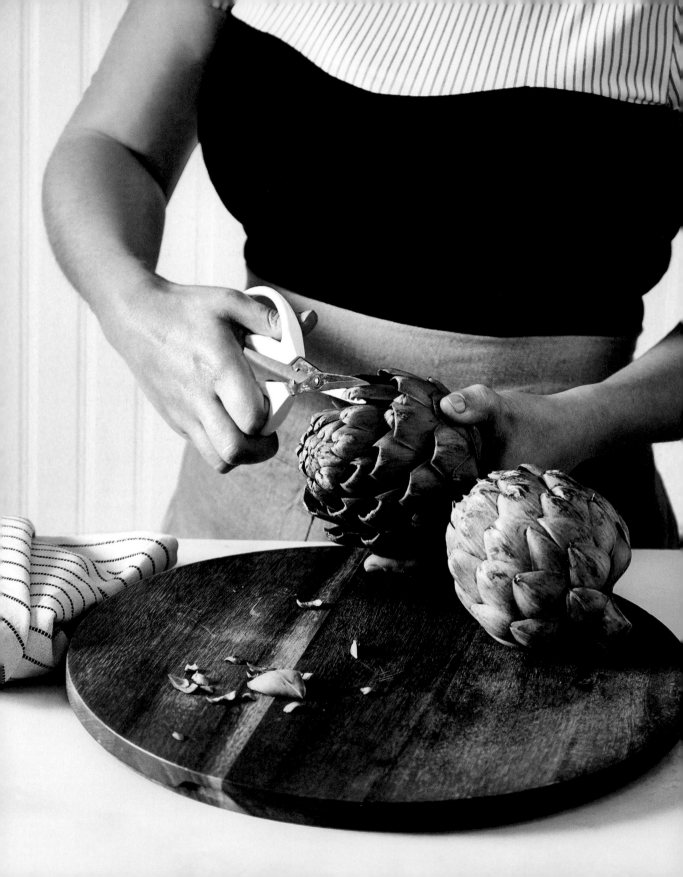

YOUR KITCHEN AIDS AND PANTRY

When you're getting started, cooking at home can be a little more time-consuming than going out, but in the end you will save money, time, and calories by cooking for yourself. And if you create a space that you love (working with what you have), you will be more inclined to stick with eating clean.

My family and I are pretty frugal. But good health is something worth investing in. And to get healthy, you need to spend a little money on tools that will set you up on the path to success. Here are some of the gadgets I recommend to help make this lifestyle sustainable in the long run. These certainly worked for me!

Important Kitchen Tools

Electric Pressure Cooker

This awesome tool is the best investment you can make. I certainly couldn't have accomplished what I did without it. A pressure cooker can take meat from frozen to cooked in a fraction of the time it would normally take to defrost and cook in a standard way. Most of the recipes in this book require or suggest the use of a multicooker that includes a pressure

cooker function. If you don't like to spend lots of time babysitting your food, this is a great investment. I use the Instant Pot because it comes with a stainless steel liner instead of a nonstick one, but there are other great multicookers on the market, as well.

At high altitudes the pressure is lower, resulting in longer cook times for most foods. If you live at a high altitude and find that your food is not cooking in the proper allotted amount of time, you should use the chart below to adjust the cook times in this book accordingly.

Cook Time Adjustments for High Altitudes

ALTITUDE	COOK TIME
3,000 ft	+5%
4,000 ft	+10%
5,000 ft	+15%
6,000 ft	+20%
7,000 ft	+25%
8,000 ft	+30%
9,000 ft	+35%
10,000 ft	+40%
11,000 ft	+45%
12,000 ft	+50%

High-Powered Blender

My first blender was a Magic Bullet. It got the job done, but within a year of every-day use I burned out the motor. Next came an Oster, then a Ninja, and finally we decided to invest in a Vitamix. High-powered blenders like the Vitamix come at a lofty price, but they will change the way you cook.

The recipes in this cookbook that call for a blender require a high-powered blender. Many of the recipes will not work with a traditional blender and could actually damage or break your blender if you do not use the correct equipment.

I use mine almost every day to make a smoothie. I also love to make batters, sauces, and dressings; the pièce de resistance is that they can blend whole grains and turn them into flour! Grinding your own flours at home is a valuable ability because as soon as the grain, seed, or nut is ground and becomes oxidized, it begins to lose some of its nutritional value. By grinding your own flours at home, you are ensuring that you get all the nutritional benefits.

Immersion Blender

For jobs big or little, an immersion blender is a super-handy kitchen tool. I love to use it to make homemade mayo, refried beans, soups, and applesauce right in the pot. It eliminates the potential for burns when transferring hot foods to a blender. I also love to use it for dressings and sauces. I put all my ingredients in a wide-mouth mason jar and blend them right in the jar!

Food Processor

I put off getting a food processor for many years, reasoning that since I already had a high-powered blender, what was a food processor going to do for me except take up precious counter space? In 2016, my husband bought me a food processor for my birthday, and now I cannot believe I'd gone without one for so many years. It's great for chopping veggies, grating cheese, or making hummus. It's a must-have in my kitchen.

Citrus Juicer

I love to start my day with a glass of lemon water. I juice one lemon with my citrus juicer and add it to 32 ounces of water. Not only does it taste delicious but it aids in detoxification. Since I love adding citrus juice to recipes, this small, handy tool is beneficial to keep around.

Juicers can range from a manual, handheld one to a stand-alone electric one. Pick the type that's right for you.

Spiralizer

One of our absolute favorite lunches is spiralized zucchini or squash with basil pesto or spaghetti sauce. I don't even bother warming the noodles because we love the raw crunch so much! Spiralizers are fun little gadgets that help replace the carb-heavy pastas in your diet. There are many to choose from, so let me save you the trouble and added expense: skip the handheld and go straight to the five-blade compact one!

Cast-Iron Skillet and Stainless Steel Pots and Pans

Cast iron can sometimes get a bad rap because it requires a different cleaning regime than typical nonstick or stainless steel pans. But there are so many videos showing you how to care for them online, which really simplify the process. I use only cast-iron or stainless steel cookware in my kitchen. Nonstick cookware contains a chemical called perfluorooctanoic acid, which can give off toxic fumes known to cause birth defects, thyroid disease, and cancer. The coating eventually breaks down over time, which means those chemicals wind up inside your food. When cooking with stainless steel and cast iron, you don't have to worry about harmful gasses or chemicals.

Strainers

There are two different strainers I use a lot in my kitchen. They both serve several purposes, from making it easier to rinse my vegetables to straining broths. I have a fine-mesh strainer for straining small things like quinoa and a stainless steel strainer that fits inside my pressure cooker to make straining beans, broths, and hard-boiled eggs easier.

Measuring Cups and Spoons

One basic set of measuring cups and spoons will provide accurate measurements, ensuring that you receive the intended results from these recipes.

Cutting Boards

I have two different types of cutting boards: wood and Dexas. The Dexas is a board made of polypropylene, ensuring it is super-durable and dishwasher safe. I use the wood cutting board for slicing fruits and vegetables that won't leave distinct flavors behind. If I'm chopping onions or cutting meats, I use the plastic board because it doesn't absorb the flavors.

Sharp Knives

A good set of knives is so important when preparing food; dull knives lead to a frustrating kitchen experience. Investing in a durable set that is able to be resharpened over time will make your kitchen prep much more enjoyable.

Glassware

I store all my food in glassware instead of plastic, so as to eliminate the potential of chemicals leaching into our foods. I love to use mason jars to store dry goods and I use them to keep fresh herbs hydrated in my refrigerator. I also use glass snapware to store leftovers.

Pantry Staples

Coconut Aminos

A soy-free substitute for soy sauce, coconut aminos is a great replacer when you start eliminating heavily processed forms of soy from your diet. This ingredient can be found near the soy sauce at the grocery store or online. Costco is even carrying it now!

Almond Flour

A great grain-free flour for a low-carbohydrate or ketogenic diet, almond flour finds its way into a lot of my dessert recipes. It's a great source of vitamin E, iron, magnesium, and calcium. This grain-free flour is an asset in any gluten-free pantry.

Coconut Flour

Coconut flour is high in protein, fiber, and healthy fats, and it has a low glycemic index. It's grain free, making it an optimal choice for those with celiac disease. (Coconut flour requires a lot more liquid in a recipe and therefore is not a great substitute for almond flour.)

Buckwheat Flour

Packed full of nutrients, this little antioxidant seed is a powerhouse! The name is deceiving, as buckwheat doesn't contain wheat at all—it's a gluten-free seed that can aid in digestion and prevent diabetes! High in fiber, nonallergenic, and great for heart health, this is one of our most beloved flours. It can be a little tricky to find in a conventional grocery store, though. I usually order mine online or pick it up at Whole Foods or Sprouts.

Coconut Sugar

A natural sweetener that's a little grittier than brown sugar, this blends well so I use it in grain-free cookies, brownies, and cakes. Coconut sugar contains a prebiotic fiber called inulin that is wonderful for digestive health and helps nourish the good bacteria in your gut.

Organic Raw Honey

Knowing where your honey comes from and how it's produced is so important. Sadly, most of the honey you find in the grocery store isn't really honey at all but, rather, made of artificial sugars and sweeteners like corn syrup. It is always best to find a local beekeeper, as local honey is a powerful aid in battling seasonal allergies and environmental ailments. If you are unable to source your honey locally, the second-best option is to find a brand that is raw, organic, and GMO free.

Coconut Palm Shortening

A blend of coconut and palm oils, this shortening is way different from Crisco! Palm oil is ideal for creating flaky baked goods, and coconut oil is nutrient-rich and packed full of health benefits from things like lauric acid, which can boost your energy and kill harmful pathogens like bacteria and viruses.

Pure Maple Syrup

The maple syrup I refer to in this cookbook is not pancake syrup. It's 100 percent pure maple syrup collected from maple trees. It takes 40 gallons of sap to make 1 gallon of maple syrup, which is why pure syrup is so pricey! Pure forms are classified as grade A and grade B, which refers to the thickness and color, not quality. They do not contain additives like high-fructose corn syrup, corn syrup, or beet sugar.

Dairy-Free Chocolate Chips

You'll see dairy-free chocolate chips referenced a lot in this cookbook. I love the Enjoy Life brand. These chocolate chips do not contain nuts, soy, or dairy products and are allergy friendly.

Almond Milk

It's so easy to make, and there's no need to pore through all the ingredients listed on the carton in the store. You can find the recipe on page 223.

Coconut Milk

We only use coconut milk from BPA-free cans, instead of the cartons in the grocery store. Those cartons usually have lots of additives and stabilizers, not to mention more water than actual coconut milk.

Ghee

Ghee is a nutty-tasting form of clarified butter; clarified butter is butter that has been heated to remove the milk solids, making it a form of dairy that is typically safe for those who have a dairy sensitivity. It is free of lactose and casein, and it can also aid in things like weight loss or improve problems with inflammation and digestion.

Brown Rice

Low in calories and rich in nutritional benefits, brown rice is a fiber-rich protein choice for anyone following a gluten-free diet. This is an important ingredient to purchase organic, as some say that organic rice has a lower arsenic content.

Quinoa

Technically not a grain, this protein-rich seed is one of the greatest sources of plant-based protein we have. This is a quality gluten-free carbohydrate to incorporate into your diet that leaves you feeling satisfied.

Sea Salt

I use sea salt or pink Himalayan salt to heighten the flavor in all my recipes. Both of these essential salts are rich in trace minerals and can help alkalize the body.

Gluten-Grain-Free Pasta

My goal is to make healthy meals that our entire family will enjoy. My three young kids really love pasta. Because we are gluten and casein free, we use alternative pastas like brown rice pasta, chickpea pasta, quinoa pasta, and black bean pasta. Ancient Harvest is our favorite brand.

Extra-Virgin Coconut Oil

This oil is a super-healthy fat that can be a great asset in a high-fat, low-carb diet. It does have saturated fat, but our bodies need some of that—at least 50 percent of our cell membranes are made up of saturated fatty acids.

Extra-Virgin Olive Oil

Full of heart-healthy macronutrients, olive oil has been a part of our diet for centuries, and there are many health benefits we can reap, from its anti-inflammatory properties to its ability to help fight cancer!

Avocado Oil

One of the healthiest oils on the planet, avocado oil has even received prescription drug status in France, owing to its ability to reduce the effects of arthritis! It can lower your cholesterol, boost nutrient absorption, and help prevent diabetes and obesity. This is a pantry must-have!

Shopping Tips

Organic Foods

When a food is labeled "100% Organic," it means the food you are consuming hasn't been treated with synthetic pesticides or insecticides. It has been grown without the use of synthetic fertilizers, sewage sludge, or ionizing radiation and doesn't contain GMOs.

This is important because when you consume nonorganic produce, you could be taking in up to thirty different types of pesticides, which are then metabolized by your body and stored in your colon. People who consume more pesticides are more likely to develop cancer, Alzheimers disease, ADHD, and have children with birth defects. These chemicals can harm the nervous system, the reproductive system, and the endocrine system.

GMOs

GMO stands for "genetically modified organism." It is suspected that consuming GMOs in large quantities can lead to infertility, gluten disorders, allergies, and even cancer.

Food Labels

Reading food labels is like learning a new language. It's not easy, but the more diligent you are at looking up the ingredients in the foods you're consuming, the easier it will become. I briefly touch on the biggest "baddies" in the labels on standard products, with the hope that it will encourage you to begin doing some research on your own. Here goes:

MSG. Monosodium glutamate is an exotoxin. It overexcites the cells in your body, stimulating them to death. Literally. It can trigger and worsen learning disabilities or Alzheimer's, and can lead to obesity. Other names for MSG are: hydrolyzed protein and vegetable protein, sodium caseinate, yeast nutrient or extract, natural flavoring, and glutamic acid.

Artificial Sweeteners. High-fructose corn syrup, dextrose, glucose, aspartame, fructose, cane juice, beet sugar, splenda/sucralose—this is not an exhaustive list. The list is long and lengthy, and these sweeteners are found not only in processed foods and desserts, where you'd expect to find them, but also in medications, children's vitamins, even toothpaste. These sweeteners are dangerous and have carcinogenic effects. They are designed by scientists to get the brain addicted to sweeteners and enslave the body to manufactured foods. Plain and simple, artificial sweeteners have no place in any home.

BHA and BHT. Butylated hydroxyanisole and butylated hydroxytoluene are preservatives commonly found in breakfast cereals and chips. They have carcinogenic properties and act as endocrine disrupters, throwing hormone production out of wack.

Soy Products. The vast majority of soy used in processed foods is genetically engineered. That means that the plant has been tinkered with at the molecular level so that it can withstand being sprayed with pesticides and other chemicals. GMO soy has some of the highest levels of glyphosate, the main ingredient in RoundUp, a common, nonselective herbicide. Not only that, but heavily processed forms of soy, like soy sauce, have been know to increase estrogen production, which in turn makes you hold on to belly fat.

Food Dyes and Additives. Red dye #40 was linked to behavioral issues and hyperactivity in children, and mice have developed tumors during testing of immune systems. Yellow dye #5 has a similar story. So, it's best to avoid dyes and artificial colors whenever possible.

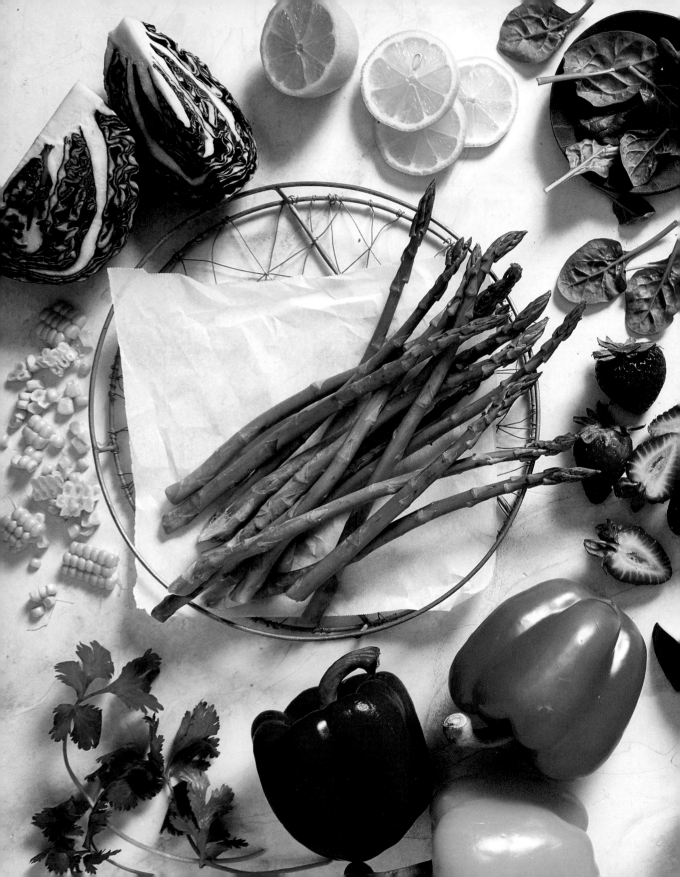

A 30-DAY MEAL PLAN

Most of my poor food choices are made at the end of the day, when I've put off making dinner or I don't have anything on the agenda. *Meal Planning is important.* The more you do it, the easier it becomes. Eventually you'll have a storehouse of favorite recipes that you know well and will keep the ingredients on hand so you'll always have a quick and easy meal to fall back on.

Here, I've presented a 30-day meal plan to get you started. Many of these meals can easily be swapped with another. Just keep in mind that you want to avoid eating two carb-heavy meals in one day. You should also drink at least eight 8-ounce glasses of water a day. And if you need a snack, you can choose from any of the vegetable side dishes or snacks in the recipe section of this book.

1

BREAKFAST:
Rainbow Juice
Smoothie

LUNCH:
Egg Salad
Lettuce Wrap

DINNER:
Skinny
Chicken
Pot Pie

2

BREAKFAST:
Coconut Flour
Pancakes

LUNCH:
Light and
Fresh
Mediterranean
Bowl

DINNER:
4-Minute
Creamy Garlic
Cauliflower
Soup

3

BREAKFAST:
Creamy Veggie
Scramble

LUNCH:
Zoodles with
Basil Pesto and
Sun-Dried
Tomatoes

DINNER:
Better than
Takeout
Orange
Chicken Bowl

4

BREAKFAST:
Blueberry
Breakfast
Cakes

LUNCH:
Honey
Mustard-
Turkey Bacon
Wrap

DINNER:
Marinated Fall-
off-the-Bone
Herb Chicken
with Savory
Bacon Brussels
Sprouts

5

BREAKFAST:
Cinnamon-
Apple Steel
Cut Oats

LUNCH:
1-Minute
Chicken Soup

DINNER:
Spaghetti
Squash with
Dairy-Free
Alfredo Sauce

6

BREAKFAST:
Chocolate PB
Oatmeal

LUNCH:
Asian Chicken
Lettuce Wrap

DINNER:
Tuscan
Chicken

7

BREAKFAST:
Instant Loss
Green Juice

LUNCH:
Cobb Salad

DINNER:
Kale and
Chicken-
Sausage
Alfredo Pizza

8

BREAKFAST:
Loaded
Breakfast
Sweet Potatoes

LUNCH:
Skinny Mac
and No Cheese

DINNER:
10-Minute
Turkey
Burgers with
leafy green
salad

9

BREAKFAST:
Coconut Milk
Yogurt with
blueberries
and granola

LUNCH:
Tuna Salad
Lettuce wrap

DINNER:
Fiery Vegan
Taco Stew

10

BREAKFAST:
Lemon Chia
Seed Muffins

LUNCH:
Simple
Chicken
Ceasar Salad

DINNER:
Egg Roll Bowl

11

BREAKFAST:
Quick Blueberry Applesauce with 1-2 Hard-Boiled Eggs

LUNCH:
Strawberry, Spinach, and Pecan Salad

DINNER:
Eggplant Parmesan

12

BREAKFAST:
Huevos Rancheros Breakfast Casserole

LUNCH:
Leftovers

DINNER:
Spicy Stuffed Peppers

13

BREAKFAST:
Chewy Cinnamon-Apple Breakfast Bars

LUNCH:
Spicy Tomato Basil Soup

DINNER:
Vegan Fajita Bowls

14

BREAKFAST:
Rainbow Juice Smoothie

LUNCH:
Summer Shrimp Scampi with Zoodles and Chickpeas

DINNER:
Shredded Beef Tacos

15

BREAKFAST:
Chicken Sausage Breakfast Salad

LUNCH:
Sun-Dried Tomato and Basil Chickpea Patties

DINNER:
Super-Simple Chili

16

BREAKFAST:
Instant Loss Green Juice

LUNCH:
Sweet and Savory Lightened-Up Chicken Salad

DINNER:
Skinny Enchiladas

17

BREAKFAST:
Savory Fried Eggs with Spinach

LUNCH:
Beef and Broccoli

DINNER:
Savory Barbecued Chicken Sliders

18

BREAKFAST:
Coconut Milk Yogurt with berries and granola

LUNCH:
Steamed Frozen Veggies

DINNER:
Veggie Fried Rice

19

BREAKFAST:
Simple Breakfast Frittata

LUNCH:
Traditional Black Bean Soup

DINNER:
Lemon Basil Salmon with Lemon Garlic-Butter Artichokes

20

BREAKFAST:
Leftovers

LUNCH:
Classic Tostadas

DINNER:
Chocolate Peanut Butter Milkshake

21

BREAKFAST:
Cranberry Orange Scones

LUNCH:
Rainbow Juice Smoothie

DINNER:
Asian Chicken Lettuce Wraps

22

BREAKFAST:
Tex-Mex Breakfast Tostadas

LUNCH:
Veggie platter with Veggie Dip: All of your favorite raw veggies, with turkey meat and Hard-Boiled Eggs

DINNER:
Fire-Roasted Beef Stew

23

BREAKFAST:
Chicken Sausage Breakfast Salad

LUNCH:
Cleaner Corn Chowder

DINNER:
Shepherd's Pie

24

BREAKFAST:
Peanut Butter Blender Mini Muffins

LUNCH:
Turkey Nuggets and Sweet Potato French Fries

DINNER:
Creamy Tuscan Chicken with Sun-Dried Tomatoes

25

BREAKFAST:
Almond Pulp Pancakes

LUNCH:
Spinach-Loaded Veggie Soup

DINNER:
Barbecued Chicken Pizza

26

BREAKFAST:
Instant Loss Green Juice

LUNCH:
Simple Chicken Ceasar Salad

DINNER:
Vegetable Lasagna

27

BREAKFAST:
Cinnamon Applesauce with Hard-Boiled Eggs

LUNCH:
Leftovers

DINNER:
Classic Meatloaf with mashed potatoes

28

BREAKFAST:
Simple Breakfast Frittata

LUNCH:
One-Pot Spaghetti with Meat Sauce

DINNER:
Zuppa Toscana

29

BREAKFAST:
Rainbow Juice Smoothie

LUNCH:
Zucchine Basilico Bowl

DINNER:
Strawberry, Spinach, and Pecan Salad

30

BREAKFAST:
Banana Chocolate Chip Blender Mini Muffins

LUNCH:
Honey Mustard–Turkey Bacon Wrap

DINNER:
Classic Pot Roast

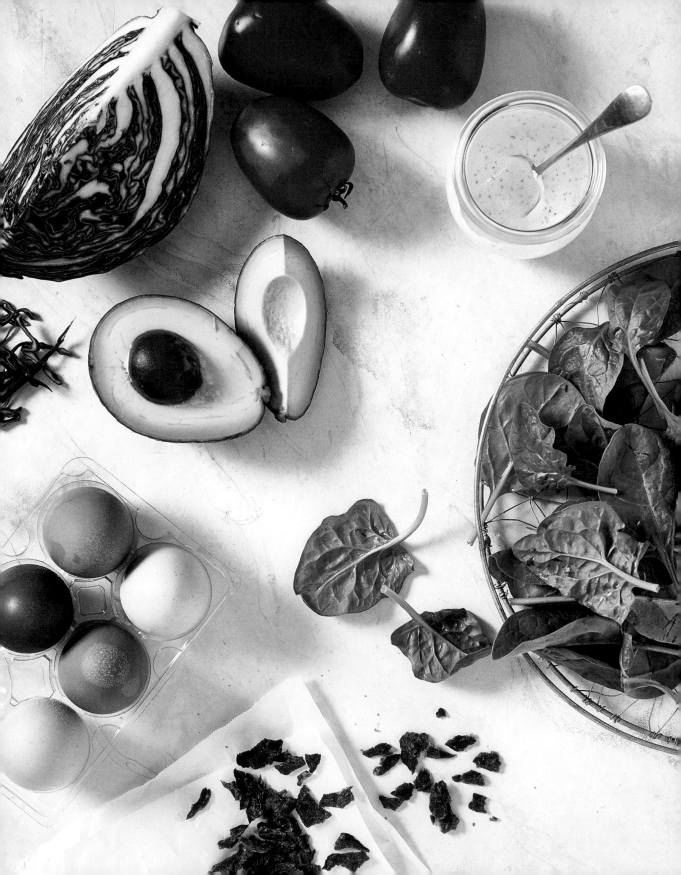

BREAKFAST
CAKES
and
MUFFINS

coconut flour *pancakes*

4 eggs

1 cup (13.5-ounce can) full-fat coconut milk or coconut cream, chilled for 8 to 12 hours

2 teaspoons pure vanilla extract

1 tablespoon organic raw honey

½ cup coconut flour

1 teaspoon baking soda

½ teaspooon sea salt

1 recipe Strawberry Syrup (page 219) or Coconut Whipped Cream (page 43)

serves 4 to 6 • **My daughter Avey's favorite breakfast has always been pancakes with whipped cream. When we were following the AIP Diet to help heal her immune system, I needed to come up with a recipe that didn't include any flour, dairy, or conventional sugar. Avey barely noticed the difference. She loved these pancakes and now the whole family does, too. They are delicious on their own or with fruit.**

1. Preheat a griddle to 350°F.

2. Crack the eggs into a medium or large bowl and whisk until frothy.

3. Thoroughly chilled, the coconut cream will separate from the liquid. Remove the cream and place back in the refrigerator (to use for the Coconut Whipped Cream topping). Measure out 1 cup of the coconut liquid and add it to the eggs.

4. Add the vanilla, honey, flour, baking soda, and salt and whisk to combine.

5. Coat the griddle with a little coconut oil or cooking spray. Use a ⅛- to ¼-cup measure to spoon some of the batter onto the griddle. Cook the pancakes on one side until lightly browned and the top begins to bubble. Flip and lightly brown on the other side. Remove the pancakes and keep warm while you make the remaining pancakes.

6. Top the pancakes with the Strawberry Syrup or Coconut Whipped Cream and serve.

grain-free *waffles*

1³/₄ cups buckwheat flour

1¹/₂ teaspoons baking powder

³/₄ teaspoon baking soda

¹/₂ teaspoon sea salt

4 eggs

2 tablespoons coconut oil

2 tablespoons organic raw honey

1 teaspoon pure vanilla extract

2 cups almond milk or water

1 teaspoon fresh lemon juice

1 recipe Strawberry Syrup
  (page 219)

1 recipe Coconut Whipped Cream
  (recipe follows)

Sliced ripe bananas and fresh
  strawberries, for serving

makes 10 waffles • **Don't let the name fool you! Buckwheat is a seed, not a grain. Not only does it lend an amazing nutty depth to the dish, it's gluten free and high in protein, amino acids, and lysine, making this a spectacular breakfast food.**

1. Preheat a waffle iron.

2. Combine the flour, baking powder, baking soda, and sea salt in a large bowl.

3. Whisk in the eggs, coconut oil, honey, vanilla, almond milk, and lemon juice.

4. Spoon about ¼ cup of batter onto the waffle iron (see manufacturer's instructions) and close to cook the waffle until crisp and brown.

5. Remove the waffle and keep warm while you make the remaining waffles. Serve with the Strawberry Syrup and the bananas and strawberries.

coconut whipped cream

makes 2 cups

1 cup chilled coconut cream

¹/₂ teaspoon pure vanilla extract

Place the chilled coconut cream in a mixer bowl. Add the vanilla. Using the whisk attachment on your hand or stand mixer, beat until the mixture forms soft peaks.

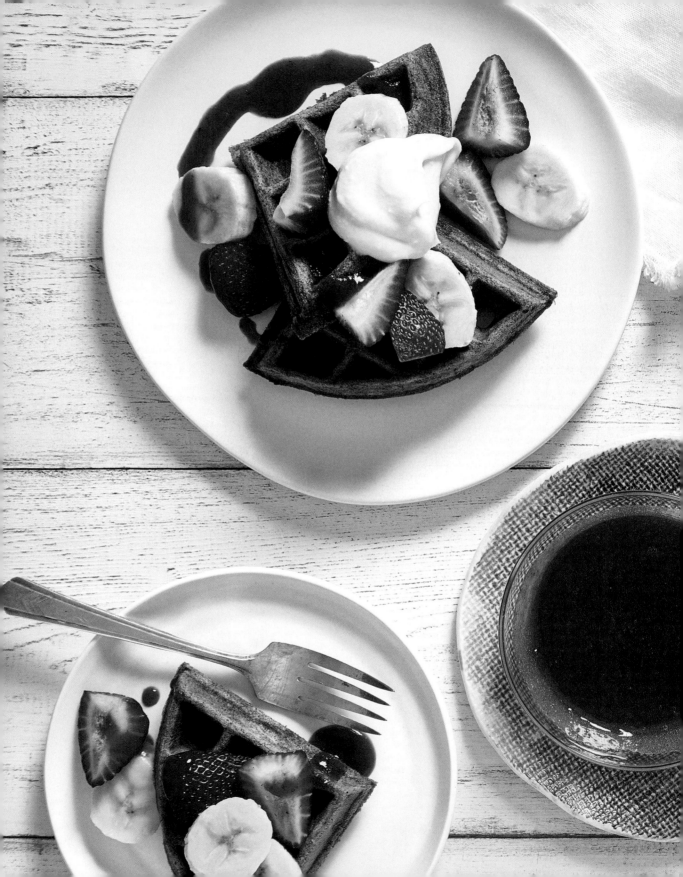

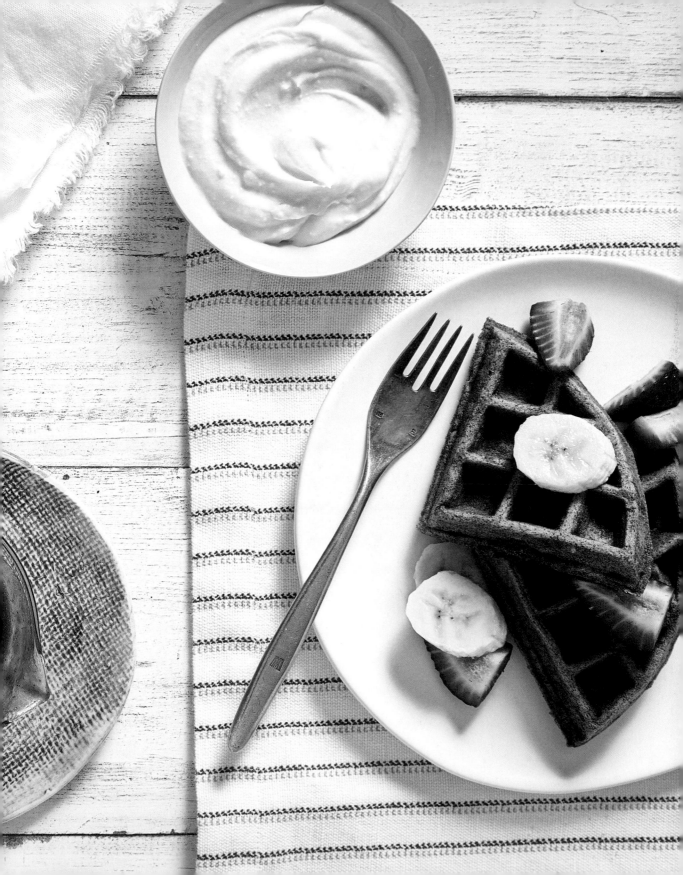

banana chocolate chip blender *mini muffins*

When we started making changes to our diet, one of the first things we did was stop eating cereal. Most cereal is very processed, full of sugar, dyes, and chemical additives that can actually be harmful to our kiddos. These little muffins made the transition so easy (and trust me, no one will be able to taste the spinach). We make them a few dozen at a time and store the remainder in the freezer. Since they're small, they take only about 15 minutes to thaw, or you can pop them in the microwave to thaw for a few seconds if you just can't wait!

2 eggs

1/3 cup organic raw honey

1/4 cup Homemade Almond Milk (page 223) or store-bought

2 tablespoons organic peanut butter, almond butter, or sunflower seed butter

3/4 cup gluten-free old-fashioned rolled oats

1 ripe banana

1 teaspoon baking soda

1 teaspoon pure vanilla extract

1 cup baby spinach (optional)

1/4 cup dairy-free mini chocolate chips (optional)

1. Preheat the oven to 350°F. Spray a 24-cup mini muffin pan with coconut oil spray.

2. Put all the ingredients, except the chocolate chips, in a high-powered blender and blend until smooth.

3. Fill the muffin cups three-fourths full. Sprinkle the tops with the chocolate chips, if using.

4. Bake for 9 to 12 minutes, or until a toothpick in the center comes out clean. Pop the muffins out of the tin and enjoy!

chewy cinnamon-apple *breakfast bars*

1 cup gluten-free quick-cooking oats

1 cup (packed) almond flour

¼ cup organic raw honey

1 egg

2 tablespoons coconut oil, solid or melted

½ teaspoon baking soda

1 teaspoon ground cinnamon

Pinch of sea salt

1 teaspoon pure vanilla extract

1 cup diced Red Delicious apple

makes 16 breakfast bars • **I have a major sweet tooth when it comes to breakfast. In particular, I'm a sucker for anything with a cinnamon-apple flavor. These delicious breakfast bars satisfy that craving, and the best part is the way they make your whole house smell like fall, all year round.**

1. Preheat the oven to 375°F. Lightly spray an 8-inch square baking pan with coconut oil spray.

2. Place all the ingredients, except the diced apple, in the bowl of a stand mixer and mix to combine (or use a hand mixer and bowl). Stir in the apple.

3. Lightly press the mixture into the prepared pan.

4. Bake for 10 to 12 minutes, or until the edges turn golden and the center is cooked through. Let cool for 15 minutes before cutting into 16 bars and serving.

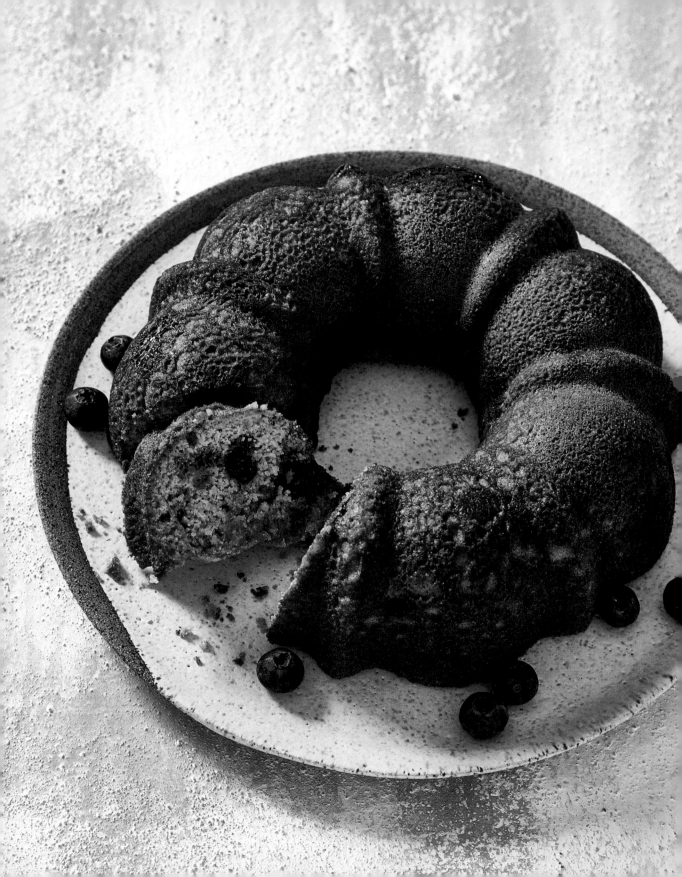

blueberry breakfast *cake*

4 eggs

⅓ cup organic raw honey

2 tablespoons avocado oil

1 teaspoon pure vanilla extract

1 cup gluten-free old-fashioned rolled oats

½ cup (packed) almond flour

2 tablespoons coconut flour

1 teaspoon baking soda

½ cup fresh blueberries

serves 6 • **Who doesn't love cake for breakfast? Baking your oats is a healthy and fun way to get all the nutritional benefits of oats and avoid the monotony of eating oatmeal every day.**

1. Preheat the oven to 350°F. Liberally coat a 6-cup Bundt or tube pan with coconut oil spray.

2. Add all the ingredients, except the blueberries, to a high-powered blender and blend on high until smooth. Stir in the blueberries by hand.

3. Pour the batter into the prepared pan.

4. Bake for 22 minutes, or until a toothpick inserted in the center of the cake comes out clean.

5. Let the cake cool for 5 minutes before turning it out onto a cake stand. Let cool and then cut into slices to serve.

tip: This cake can also be made in a pressure cooker. Pour the batter into the prepared pan and cover with foil. Pour about 1 cup water into the pressure cooker. Put the cake pan on the trivet and gently lower it into the cooker. Place the lid on the cooker and set the vent valve to SEALING position. Using the display panel, select the MANUAL/PRESSURE COOK function, high pressure, and use the +/- buttons until the display reads 30 minutes. When the cooking time is up, do a quick release, moving the pressure knob from the SEALING to the VENTING position. Using caution, open the cooker and lift the cake pan out. Let the cake cool for 5 minutes and remove the foil before turning it out onto a cake stand.

peanut butter blender *mini muffins*

makes 24 mini muffins • **This recipe uses a nut or seed butter as the "flour" base. I didn't trust this idea at first, but my mom tried it and convinced me to give it a go. It's brilliant, because the nut butter's oil content makes the resulting muffin so much more moist. My kids went crazy for her muffins, so I adapted her recipe and came up with these scrumptious minis. I say breakfast, but they really taste more like dessert to me!**

1 ripe banana

3 tablespoons organic raw honey

1 tablespoon pure vanilla extract

1 egg

1 teaspoon cacao powder

¼ teaspoon baking soda

Pinch of sea salt

½ cup organic peanut butter or nut/seed butter of choice

½ cup baby spinach

3 tablespoons dairy-free mini chocolate chips (optional)

1. Preheat the oven to 400°F. Spray a 24-cup mini muffin pan liberally with coconut oil spray.

2. Add all the ingredients, except the chocolate chips, to a high-powered blender. Blend on high until smooth.

3. Fill the cups half to three-fourths full and sprinkle the tops with the chocolate chips, if using.

4. Bake for 7 to 9 minutes, or until the muffin centers are cooked through. Pop them out of the tin and enjoy!

lemon chia seed *muffins*

1 cup coconut flour

½ teaspoon sea salt

1 teaspoon baking soda

½ cup plus 2 tablespoons organic raw honey

½ cup canned coconut milk, room temperature

½ cup fresh lemon juice

¼ cup grated lemon zest

6 eggs, room temperature

1 tablespoon pure vanilla extract

¼ cup extra-virgin coconut oil, melted

¼ cup chia seeds

makes 18 muffins • **My grandma makes the most amazing lemon cake. Brady calls it Lemon Zinger Cake because it tastes just like those Little Debbie snacks. Using my grandma's cake as inspiration, I came up with this recipe that is way lower in calories! While Brady might be able to tell the difference, no one else can. If you love lemons, this one is for you!**

1. Preheat the oven to 350°F. Line a standard 12-cup muffin pan with paper or silicone liners.

2. Sift the coconut flour, sea salt, and baking soda into a small bowl.

3. In a large bowl, combine the honey, coconut milk, lemon juice, lemon zest, eggs, vanilla, and coconut oil. Add the chia seeds, and using a hand mixer, blend on low until smooth. Let the mixture sit for 10 minutes.

4. Pour the flour mixture into the batter and mix well.

5. Fill the muffin cups three-fourths full.

6. Bake for 25 to 30 minutes, or until the muffins are golden and a toothpick inserted in the center comes out clean. Turn out to cool on a rack.

7. Repeat with the remaining batter to make the rest of the muffins.

cranberry orange *scones*

2¼ cups (packed) almond flour

½ teaspoon sea salt

½ teaspoon baking soda

2 eggs

¼ cup agave nectar

⅓ cup avocado oil

1 tablespoon grated orange zest

½ cup dried cranberries

makes about 20 to 24 scones • **Scones are a favorite in our house, perfect with coffee or tea in the morning. The almond flour and avocado oil increases the nutritional value. One day, Avey suggested adding cranberries with a little orange zest, and this version was born. You can also substitute chocolate chips for the cranberries and orange zest, or fresh diced strawberries for a refreshing take.**

1. Preheat the oven to 350°F. Spray a cookie sheet with coconut oil spray.

2. Place all the ingredients in a bowl and stir with a spoon until well combined.

3. Use a cookie scoop to form balls with the batter and place them on the cookie sheet. You can place them close together, as they don't spread much. The batter should yield 20 to 24 scones.

4. Bake for 9 to 12 minutes, or until golden brown on the bottom.

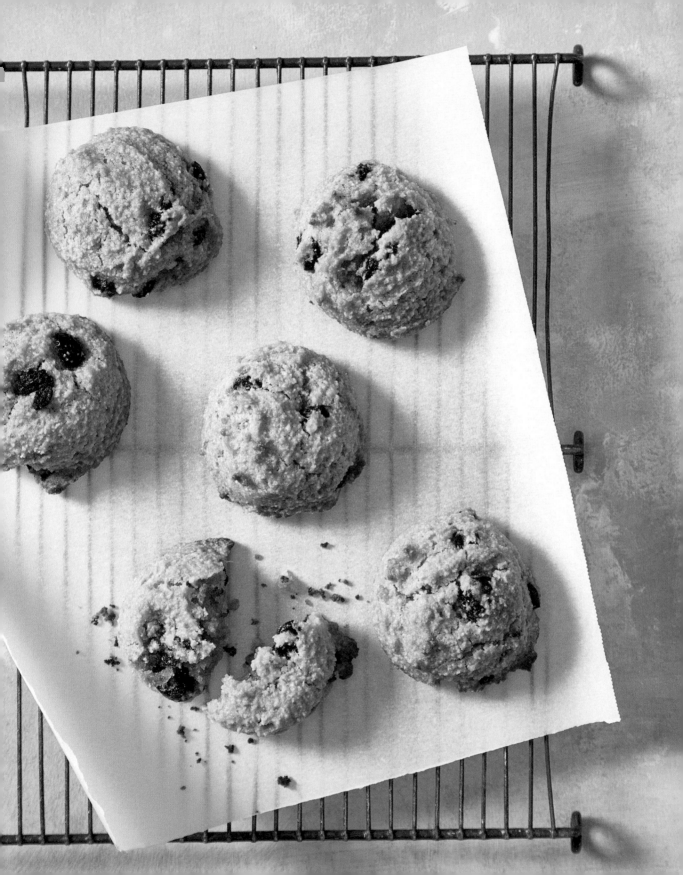

grain-free banana bread

½ cup coconut sugar

1 cup (packed) almond flour

½ cup coconut flour

1 tablespoon avocado oil

2 eggs

½ tablespoon pure vanilla extract

½ teaspoon baking soda

½ teaspoon sea salt

2 large ripe bananas

⅓ cup walnuts or pecans, chopped

makes 1 loaf • **Ever notice how kids won't go near a banana that's overripe? For this recipe, the more brown spots they have, the better. Super-ripe bananas make for delicious and sweet banana bread. The fact that this recipe is also AIP-compliant means that everyone can enjoy it!**

1. Preheat the oven to 350°F. Liberally spray a 9 by 5-inch loaf pan with coconut oil spray.

2. Place all the ingredients, except the walnuts, in a food processor, liquids first, and blend until smooth. Stir in the walnuts.

3. Pour the batter into the loaf pan and smooth the top.

4. Bake for 35 to 40 minutes, or until a toothpick inserted in the center comes out clean.

5. Let cool for about 5 minutes and then turn out onto a rack to cool completely.

almond pulp *pancakes*

1½ cups almond pulp, leftover from Homemade Almond Milk (page 223)

4 eggs

¼ cup Homemade Almond Milk (page 223) or store-bought

1 tablespoon organic raw honey

2 teaspoons pure vanilla extract

1 teaspoon baking soda

¼ teaspoon sea salt

Coconut oil (solid), for serving

1 recipe Strawberry Syrup (page 219), for serving

makes 16 to 18 small pancakes • **I'm the oldest of seven kids. Letting food go to waste was not okay in our household. When I started making my own almond milk, so many of the recipes online said to throw away the leftover almond pulp. Almonds are expensive, ya'll! This is a no-waste recipe. Here's a way to use all the almond pulp leftover from making Homemade Almond Milk (page 223), turning your "trash" into treasure!**

1. Preheat a griddle. Spray the griddle with coconut oil spray.

2. Place all the ingredients, except the coconut oil and Strawberry Syrup, in a high-powered blender. Blend on high until smooth.

3. Use a ¼ cup measure to ladle some batter onto the griddle. Cook the pancakes until air bubbles begin to form on top and the bottom is lightly browned. (Note: Almond flour gets darker more quickly than regular flour so don't be alarmed if your pancakes are very dark.)

4. Flip the pancakes and cook for another 3 to 5 minutes. Remove from the griddle and keep warm while you make the remaining pancakes.

5. To serve, spread the pancakes with coconut oil and drizzle with the Strawberry Syrup.

HEARTY BREAKFASTS

instant loss
green juice

1 cup water

½ lemon, juiced (about
   2 tablespoons)

½ green or red apple

1 cup baby spinach

½ cup chopped kale

2 tablespoons diced cucumber

½ cup sliced strawberries

serves 1 • **I love to start my mornings with a smoothie. You can sneak a lot of vegetables into this one meal. I began adding the lemon juice because lemons are great for detoxing, but if you're not as into lemons as I am, you can certainly cut the lemon here to 1 teaspoon. Your smoothie will taste just as good.**

Place all the ingredients in a high-powered blender and blend until smooth.

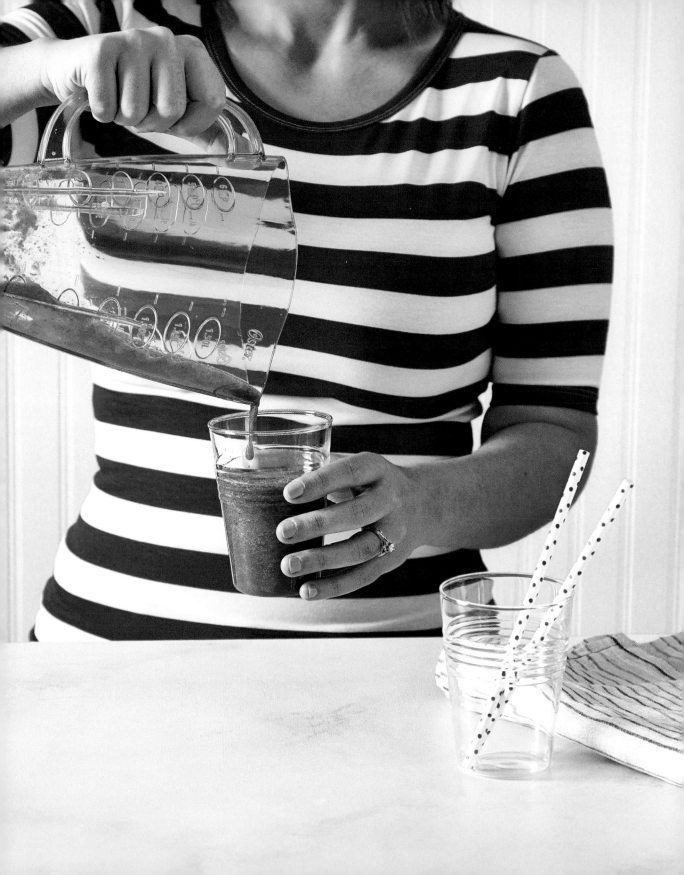

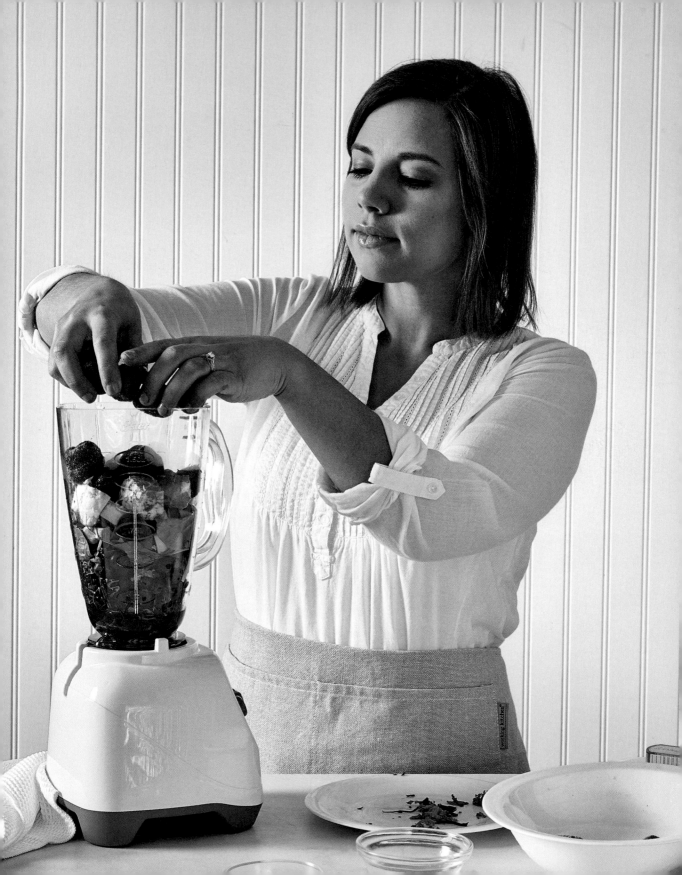

rainbow juice *smoothie*

serves 4 • Rainbows are important in our house. This is one of my kids' favorite smoothies. They help place all the fruits and veggies into the blender in the order given here (and the order matters to achieve the best consistency!). Red, orange, yellow, green, blue, and purple—and then we watch all those gorgeous colors create something new.

1½ cups water

1 lemon, juiced (about ¼ cup)

1 cup frozen strawberries

½ cup blueberries, fresh or frozen

1 orange, peeled

½ cup diced cucumber

½ cup shredded red cabbage

1 cup baby spinach

½ cup chopped kale

1 tablespoon coconut oil (optional)

1 teaspoon whole golden flaxseed (optional)

Place all the ingredients in a high-powered blender. Blend on high until the mixture is liquid smooth.

loaded breakfast sweet potatoes

2 small to medium unpeeled sweet
  potatoes

2 tablespoons pure maple syrup

1 tablespoon unsweetened
  Homemade Almond Milk
  (page 223) or store-bought

1 teaspoon ground cinnamon

4 slices turkey bacon, cooked and
  crumbled

¼ cup chopped pecans or walnuts

¼ cup blueberries, fresh or frozen (if
  frozen, thaw before using)

serves 2 to 4 • **This sweet potato breakfast is a delicious way to begin your morning with complex carbs and a good dose of protein. Sweet potatoes are high in beta-carotene, which converts to vitamin A in the body and helps boost immune function.**

1. Using a fork, poke holes all over the potatoes.

2. Pour about 1 cup water into a pressure cooker. Place the trivet or steamer basket inside the pot and set the sweet potatoes on top.

3. Place the lid on the pot and make sure the pressure knob is in the SEALING position. Using the display panel, select the MANUAL/ PRESSURE COOK function for high pressure, and use the +/- buttons until the display reads 16 minutes.

4. Combine the maple syrup, almond milk, and cinnamon in a bowl.

5. When the cooker beeps to let you know it's finished, let it naturally come down from pressure until the display reads LO:15. Switch the pressure knob from the SEALING to the VENTING position. Use caution while the steam escapes—it's hot.

6. Open the cooker and carefully remove the potatoes. Slice the potatoes open and top with the turkey bacon, pecans, blueberries, and maple syrup dressing. Serve warm.

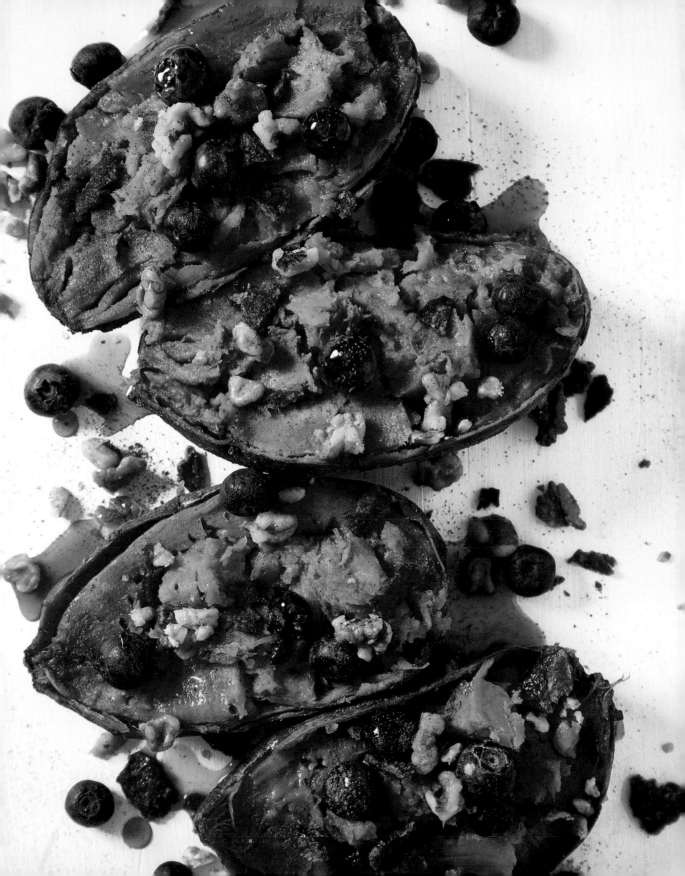

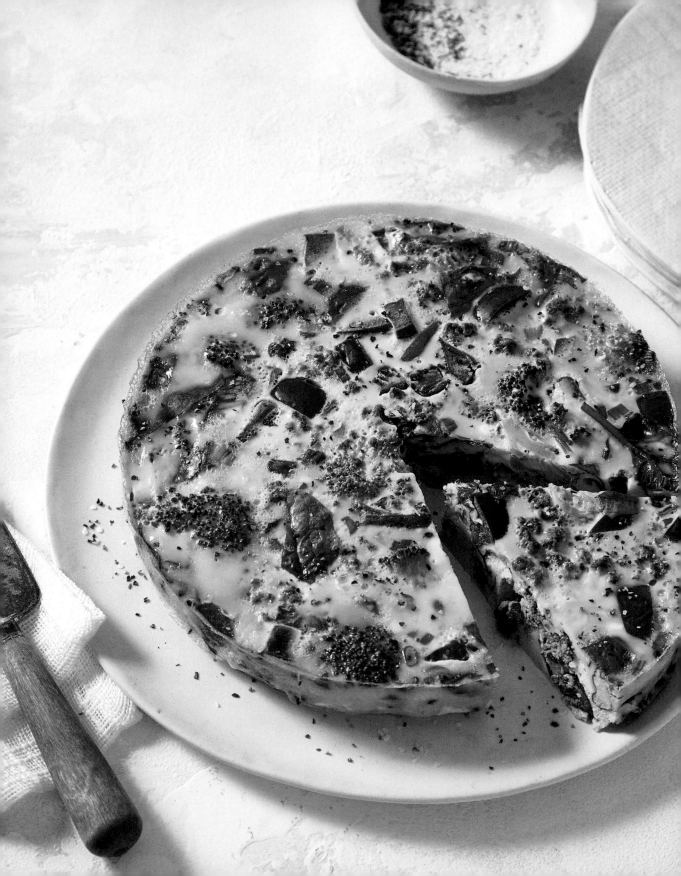

simple breakfast *frittata*

½ cup diced broccoli florets

½ cup chopped baby spinach

½ cup diced ripe tomato

8 eggs

2 tablespoons Homemade Almond Milk (page 223) or store-bought

1 tablespoon diced green onion

½ teaspoon sea salt

¼ teaspoon black pepper

½ cup cooked ground beef or sausage (optional)

serves 4 to 6 • **The sky is the limit when making a frittata. Throw in all your leftover veggies, and you'll have a filling and healthy breakfast. I also love to add leftover taco meat, but you can add any leftover meat you have in the fridge. Why let it go to waste when you can put it in a frittata?**

1. Coat with cooking spray a 3- to 6-cup baking dish that fits inside your pressure cooker.

2. Layer the broccoli, spinach, and tomato in the dish.

3. Crack the eggs into a bowl and whisk with the almond milk, green onion, salt, and pepper. Pour on top of the vegetable layer. Sprinkle on the meat, if using.

4. Cover the pan with foil and place on top of the trivet.

5. Pour about 1 cup water into the cooker and carefully lower the trivet and dish into the pot.

6. Place the lid on the cooker and make sure the pressure knob is in the SEALING position. Using the display panel, select the MANUAL/PRESSURE COOK function, high pressure, and use the +/- buttons until the display reads 30 minutes.

7. When the cooker beeps to let you know it's finished, switch the pressure knob from the SEALING to the VENTING position, administering a quick release. Use caution while the steam escapes—it's hot.

8. Open the cooker and remove the frittata. Serve warm.

savory fried eggs with spinach

1 tablespoon avocado oil or olive oil

2 eggs

Sea salt

Black pepper

½ Roma (plum) tomato, diced

1 large handful of baby spinach

1 to 2 green onions, diced

1 tablespoon chopped fresh cilantro

serves 1 • **So simple. So filling. During the year that I lost over 100 pounds, my breakfast was usually an Instant Loss Green Juice (page 58) or this fried egg recipe. Keeping it simple kept me on track. So if you're feeling overwhelmed, remember: just keep it simple.**

1. Preheat a skillet over medium-low heat and add the avocado oil. Add the eggs and fry with a sprinkling of salt and pepper to desired doneness, then remove from the skillet and place on a serving plate.

2. Add the tomato, spinach, and green onions to the pan. Sauté until the spinach wilts.

3. Top the eggs with the tomato-spinach mixture. Sprinkle with additional salt and pepper, and the cilantro.

creamy veggie scramble

2 tablespoons avocado oil

1/2 pound small sweet potatoes, cubed

1/2 red bell pepper, diced

1/2 medium onion, diced

3 white button mushrooms, thinly sliced

1 teaspoon sea salt

1/2 teaspoon dried oregano

1/2 teaspoon dried basil

1/4 teaspoon red pepper flakes

1 cup baby spinach

6 eggs, cracked and whisked in a bowl

1/4 teaspoon black pepper

serves 4 to 6 • **This flavorful, creamy egg dish will leave you feeling full all morning long while also giving you healthy servings of veggies to start your day. If you slice the veggies the night before and store them in an airtight container in the refrigerator, your prep time will be cut down to almost nothing and you can spend more time sleeping!**

1. Preheat the pressure cooker using the SAUTE function. When the display panel reads HOT, add the avocado oil, sweet potatoes, bell pepper, onion, mushrooms, 1/2 teaspoon of the salt, the oregano, basil, and red pepper flakes to the pot. Sauté for 10 minutes or until the veggies begin to become tender.

2. Smooth the vegetables out into a single layer on the bottom of the pot. Layer 1 cup of spinach over, then pour in the eggs and season with the remaining 1/2 teaspoon salt and the pepper.

3. Place the lid on the pot and make sure the pressure knob is in the SEALING position. Using the display panel, press the CANCEL button, then select the STEAM function, high pressure, and use the +/- buttons until the display reads 4 minutes.

4. When the cooker beeps to let you know it's finished, switch the pressure knob from the SEALING to the VENTING position, causing a quick pressure release. Use caution while the steam escapes—it's hot.

5. Remove the lid and stir the scramble with a wooden spoon. Serve warm.

chicken sausage *breakfast* salad

1 tablespoon extra-virgin olive oil

2 chicken sausages, sliced into
 ¼-inch pieces

⅓ cup diced red bell pepper

⅓ cup diced button mushrooms

½ teaspoon dried basil

½ teaspoon dried oregano

1 cup chopped kale

2 cups baby spinach

serves 4 • **When you're trying to cut down the amount of sugar in your diet, it's a good idea to avoid it in all forms for a while. Breakfast salad may sound counterintuitive, but I promise you: starting your day with this savory mix of veggies, chicken sausage, and herbs will leave you feeling energized. It's a great way to keep the sugar bug at bay.**

1. Heat a skillet over medium heat. When warm, add the olive oil, sausage, bell pepper, mushrooms, basil, and oregano. Sauté until the vegetables soften and the sausage begins to brown, about 5 minutes. Add the kale and cook until wilted.

2. Serve on a bed of raw baby spinach.

huevos rancheros *breakfast casserole*

1 ripe tomato, diced

½ jalapeño, diced

½ medium onion, diced

¼ cup fresh cilantro, finely chopped

1 garlic clove, diced

½ lime, juiced

1 teaspoon ground cumin

¼ teaspoon sea salt

¼ teaspoon chili powder

Extra-virgin olive oil

9 organic corn tortillas

1 cup cooked black beans, homemade (page 226) or canned, rinsed and drained

8 eggs

serves 4 to 6 • **This yummy eggy breakfast casserole can be baked in the oven (350°F for 15 minutes) or in a pressure cooker!**

1. Put the tomato, jalapeño, onion, cilantro, garlic, lime juice, cumin, salt, and chili powder in a blender or food processor and pulse until it looks like chunky salsa.

2. Coat a 6-cup baking dish with olive oil.

3. Tear 3 tortillas into fourths. Layer the bottom of the dish with the tortillas. Spoon about one-fourth of the salsa mixture and one-third of the beans over the tortillas.

4. Crack 2 eggs and gently place on top of the salsa and bean mixture on opposite sides.

5. Repeat the layering two more times. On the final layer, add the remaining 2 eggs for a total of 4 eggs on top.

6. Cover the dish with foil and place on the trivet. Pour about 1 cup water into the cooker and carefully lower the trivet and dish into the pot.

7. Place the lid on the pot and make sure the pressure knob is in the SEALING position. Using the display panel, select the MANUAL/PRESSURE COOK function, high pressure, and use the +/- buttons until the display reads 7 minutes.

8. When the cooker beeps to let you know it's finished, let it naturally come down from pressure until the display reads LO:5. Switch the pressure knob from the SEALING to the VENTING position. Use caution while the steam escapes—it's hot.

9. Remove the lid and lift out the casserole. Serve immediately.

tex-mex breakfast tostadas

serves 4 • **Tostadas are an amazing meal for families that have picky eaters or preferences that vary. I like to place all the ingredients in separate bowls and let my kiddos build their tostadas to their preference. No complaining AND it makes them feel more grown up.**

3 tablespoons avocado oil

4 organic 6-inch corn tortillas

1 cup cooked black beans, homemade (page 226) or canned, rinsed and drained

1 teaspoon taco seasoning, homemade (page 231) or store-bought

6 eggs

1 tablespoon water

Sea salt

Black pepper

1/2 cup salsa of choice

1/2 avocado, diced

2 tablespoons chopped fresh cilantro

1. Heat a skillet over medium heat. When warm, add 1 tablespoon of the oil and warm each side of the tortillas. Remove and keep warm.

2. Add the beans, taco seasoning, and another tablespoon oil to the pan. Sauté and lightly mash the beans, then transfer to a bowl. Cover and keep warm.

3. Crack the eggs into a bowl and add the water. Whisk until frothy.

4. Add the remaining tablespoon oil to the skillet and add the eggs. Lightly season with salt and pepper. When the edges of the eggs begin to set, push the sides to the center and scramble.

5. Place the beans on top of the warm tortillas and top with some egg, salsa, avocado, and cilantro.

peanut butter chocolate *oatmeal*

2 tablespoons ghee or extra-virgin coconut oil

1 heaping tablespoon cacao powder

Pinch of sea salt

1 cup gluten-free old-fashioned rolled oats

2½ cups water

¼ cup plus 1 tablespoon pure maple syrup

2 tablespoons creamy peanut, almond, or sunflower seed butter

serves 4 • **This is my favorite oatmeal—in the history of forever. You know how Cocoa Pebbles taste after they soak in milk for a little while? This oatmeal tastes just like that, with a peanut butter flair. If you can't have nut or seed butters, omit it for a cocoa oatmeal treat!**

1. Place the ghee, cacao powder, salt, oats, and water in a pressure cooker.

2. Place the lid on the pot. Make sure the pressure knob is in the SEALING position. Using the display panel, select the MANUAL/PRESSURE COOK function, high pressure, and use the +/- buttons until the display reads 8 minutes.

3. When the cooker beeps to let you know it's finished, switch the pressure knob from the SEALING to the VENTING position, causing a quick pressure release. Use caution while the steam escapes—it's hot.

4. Stir in the maple syrup and the nut butter. Serve warm.

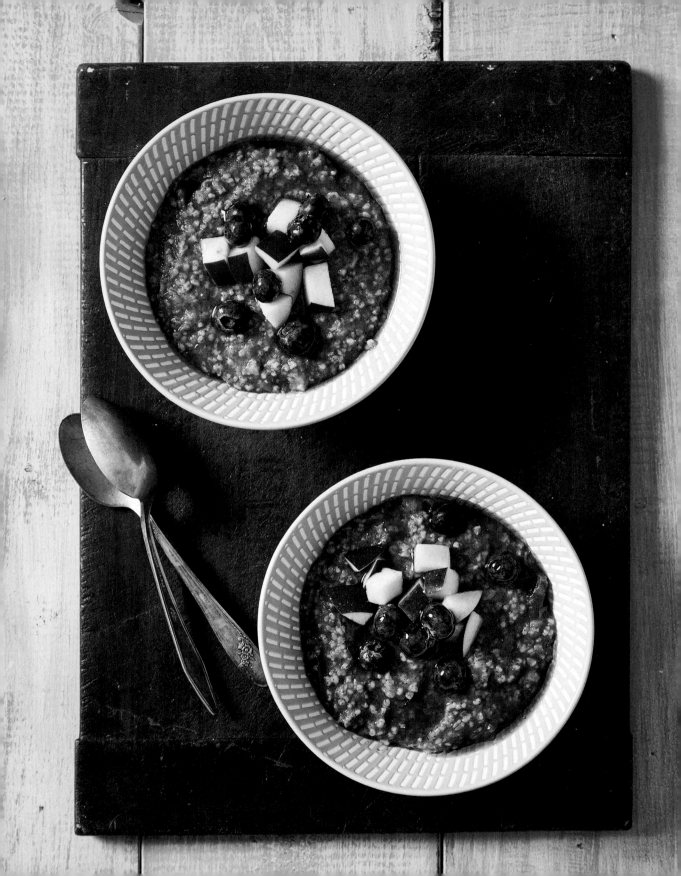

cinnamon-apple steel cut oats

2 tablespoons extra-virgin coconut oil

2 red apples, cored and diced

2 teaspoons ground cinnamon

Pinch of sea salt

1/2 cup steel cut oats

1 1/2 cups water

2 tablespoons pure maple syrup

serves 4 • **My husband is the oatmeal guy (in addition to being the love of my life), and this is an adaptation of one of his recipes. Every Saturday morning he gets up early with the kiddos so that I can work in peace. (See what I mean about love of my life?) He always makes a batch of steel cut oats, but he's forever experimenting with different flavor profiles (strawberry preserves, peaches and coconut cream, and peanut butter chocolate, which is on page 71). Apple-cinnamon girl that I am, this is one of my favorites.**

1. Preheat the pressure cooker using the SAUTE function. When the display panel reads HOT, add the oil, apples, cinnamon, and salt. Using a wooden spoon, sauté for 2 minutes.

2. As the apples begin to become tender, add the oats and sauté to lightly toast them, another minute or two.

3. Add the water and place the lid on the pot. Make sure the pressure knob is in the SEALING position. Using the display panel, select the MANUAL/PRESSURE COOK function, high pressure, and use the +/- buttons until the display reads 12 minutes.

4. When the cooker beeps to let you know it's finished, switch the pressure knob from the SEALING to the VENTING position, causing a quick pressure release. Use caution while the steam escapes—it's hot.

5. Remove the lid and stir in the maple syrup. The oats will thicken and absorb more water as they cool. Serve warm.

coconut milk *yogurt*

2 (13.5-ounce) cans full-fat coconut milk or coconut cream

2 teaspoons to 1 tablespoon grass-fed beef unflavored gelatin

2 tablespoons pure maple syrup

2 probiotic capsules (I like to use Renew Life brand)

1 vanilla bean (optional)

serves 8 • One of my favorite things to eat in the morning is yogurt. We used to eat Greek yogurt mixed with delicious strawberry preserves, but when we began to weed out dairy, yogurt was among the first items to go. It was then that I began experimenting with coconut milk. This recipe will last up to a week in the refrigerator and is a great substitute for dairy yogurt, even with its slight coconut taste (or perhaps because of it).

1. Place the coconut milk in a pressure cooker or yogurt maker and whisk until smooth.

2. Using the display panel, select the YOGURT function. Using the ADJUST button, program the pot to BOIL. This is going to warm the milk, about 15 minutes.

3. When the time has passed, use a kitchen thermometer to check the temperature of the milk. It needs to be heated to 180°F to kill any harmful bacteria. If the milk is not hot enough, press the SAUTE function until the screen reads MORE. Stir constantly while the milk heats to the appropriate temperature.

4. Once the milk has reached 180°F, carefully remove the liner of the pressure cooker that contains the milk to stop the cooking process. Ladle out ⅓ cup hot milk into a separate container and stir in the gelatin and maple syrup. Pour the mixture back into the milk and stir well until fully incorporated. (Note: The maple syrup must be added, as it is what feeds the probiotic.)

5. Transfer the milk to a container and let cool to 90 to 100°F, usually about 25–30 minutes. This ensures the heat will not kill the probiotic culture. When it has cooled, open the probiotic capsules and add the powder. Whisk.

6. Place the milk back into the pressure cooker and select the YOGURT function, NORMAL. Use the ADUST button and set the time to 8 hours. The longer you leave it in the pot, the more tart the yogurt will become. Place the lid on the pressure cooker. It does not matter if you seal it or not, it will not come to pressure.

7. When the yogurt is done culturing, it will have thickened slightly but still be very runny. If using vanilla, scrape out the seeds from the pod and into the yogurt.

8. Transfer the yogurt to a glass container, lay a sheet of plastic wrap directly over the yogurt to prevent a crust from forming, and refrigerate overnight or for a minimum of 4 hours while the yogurt thickens.

tip: The amount of gelatin you use will dictate the thickness of the yogurt. Start with 2 teaspoons and if it's not as thick as you prefer, add a little more next time.

quick blueberry applesauce

1 large red apple, cored and cubed

½ cup blueberries, fresh or frozen

2 teaspoons fresh lemon juice

makes 2 cups • **If your children are at all like mine, they're ravenous, bottomless food pits. It's always nice to be able to throw a couple things into the blender and fix them a healthy snack. This applesauce is as easy as pie (easier, really)—just three simple ingredients. You can rest assured that this snack is a good one for little tummies.**

Place the apple, blueberries, and lemon juice in a high-powered blender. Process to desired thickness, chunky or smooth. (The sauce will keep in the refrigerator for 5 days.)

classic cinnamon applesauce

makes 2 quarts • **Did you know that apple skins contain most of the fruit's vitamins and nutrients? I like to leave the skins on our apples when I make our homemade applesauce. If you prefer chunky applesauce, remove the skins and mash the apple with a potato masher instead of blending.**

1/4 cup fresh lemon juice

5 pounds red apples, cored

1 tablespoon ground cinnamon

1. Place the lemon juice, apples, and cinnamon in a pressure cooker.

2. Put the lid on the pot and make sure the pressure knob is in the SEALING position. Using the display panel, select the MANUAL/PRESSURE COOK function, high pressure, and use the +/- buttons until the display reads 5 minutes.

3. When the cooker beeps to let you know it's finished, let it naturally come down from pressure until the display reads LO:30. Switch the pressure knob from the SEALING to the VENTING position. Use caution while the steam escapes—it's hot.

4. Use an immersion blender to puree the apple mixture or very carefully transfer to a high-powered blender and blend on high until smooth. (The sauce can be stored in the refrigerator for 7 to 10 days, or freeze for up to 6 months.)

CHILIS, SOUPS, and STEWS

1-minute chicken soup

serves 4 to 6 • **Chicken soup is one of my favorite "throw it all in the pot" low-carb meals. You can add so many different kinds of vegetables (here's how to use up your leftovers!) and seasonings to vary this basic recipe. And to top it all, it takes only one pressure-cooking minute!**

2½ cups chicken broth, homemade (page 220) or store-bought

2 cups diced cooked and seasoned chicken

1 cup diced carrots (about 2 medium)

1 cup diced celery (about 2 stalks)

1 medium onion, diced

½ tablespoon dried parsley

½ tablespoon dried minced onion

½ tablespoon garlic powder

Pinch of red pepper flakes

Sea salt

1. Place all the ingredients in a pressure cooker.

2. Place the lid on the cooker and make sure the pressure knob is in the SEALING position. Using the display panel, select the MANUAL function, high pressure, and use the +/- buttons until the display reads 1 minute.

3. When the cooker beeps to let you know it's finished, switch the pressure knob from the SEALING to the VENTING position, administering a quick release. Use caution while the steam escapes—it's hot.

4. Remove the lid and serve.

fiery vegan *taco stew*

1 large onion, diced

1 large red bell pepper, cored and diced

1 to 2 jalapeños, diced (seeds and ribs removed if you like it less spicy)

4 cups vegetable broth, homemade (page 221) or store-bought

5 garlic cloves, finely chopped

1 tablespoon ground cumin

1 teaspoon cayenne (optional)

1¼ teaspoons sea salt, plus more to taste

1 (16-ounce) package lentils

1 (15-ounce) can organic diced tomatoes

¼ cup chopped fresh cilantro

1 avocado, diced

serves 6 to 8 • **Spices! Spices! Spices! This fiery stew gives a one-two punch. The cilantro aids in detoxing the body and lowering blood pressure, and the garlic combats sickness. With its mix of veggies and protein-packed lentils, this is a complete, filling meal.**

1. Preheat the pressure cooker using the SAUTE function. When the display panel reads HOT, add the onion, bell pepper, and jalapeño. Cook, stirring frequently, until the vegetables brown and begin to stick to the bottom of the pot, about 6 minutes.

2. Stir in 2 tablespoons of the broth and continue to cook, stirring, until the onion is soft and lightly browned, another 5 minutes.

3. Stir in the garlic, cumin, cayenne (if using), and salt. Cook for 1 minute, stirring constantly. Add the lentils, tomatoes, and remaining broth.

4. Place the lid on the cooker and make sure the pressure knob is in the SEALING position. Using the display panel, press the CANCEL button, then select the MANUAL/PRESSURE COOK function, high pressure, and use the +/- buttons until the display reads 10 minutes.

5. When the cooker beeps to let you know it's finished, let it naturally come down from pressure until the display reads LO:10. Switch the pressure knob from the SEALING to the VENTING position. Use caution while the steam escapes—it's hot.

6. Serve with the cilantro and avocado, adjusting the salt to taste.

spicy tomato basil soup

2 tablespoons olive oil

1 large onion, diced

½ cup diced celery
(about 1 stalk)

1 cup diced carrots
(about 2 medium)

1 teaspoon sea salt

½ teaspoon black pepper

¼ teaspoon red pepper flakes

½ cup chopped fresh basil

2 dried bay leaves

2 (15-ounce) cans organic
diced tomatoes

2 cups vegetable broth,
homemade (page 221)
or store-bought

½ cup full-fat coconut milk

Grain-Free Garlic Biscuits
(page 185; optional)

serves 6 • Tomato soup with grilled cheese was one of my favorite autumn lunches before I got serious about health. When I started reading the ingredients, I realized that my beloved tomato soup contained absolutely everything I should NOT be eating: high-fructose corn syrup, wheat, dairy, and tons of preservatives. While it's not as easy as just opening a can of soup, this homemade soup is pretty simple and full of flavor. Instead of eating it with grilled cheese, I like it served with a side of my Grain-Free Garlic Biscuits (page 185). And if the soup is too spicy for you, feel free to leave out the red pepper flakes.

1. Preheat the pressure cooker using the SAUTE function. When the display panel reads HOT, add the oil to the pot and saute the onion, celery, and carrots until they begin to soften, about 5 minutes.

2. Add the salt, pepper, red pepper flakes, basil, bay leaves, tomatoes, broth, and coconut milk to the pot.

3. Place the lid on the cooker and make sure the pressure knob is in the SEALING position. Using the display panel, press the CANCEL button, then select the MANUAL/PRESSURE COOK function, high pressure, and use the +/- buttons until the display reads 5 minutes.

4. When the cooker beeps to let you know it's finished, let it naturally come down from pressure until the display reads LO:10. Switch the pressure knob from the SEALING to the VENTING position. Use caution while the steam escapes—it's hot.

5. Remove the bay leaves and blend the soup with an immersion blender. Serve warm with the biscuits, if desired.

zuppa toscana

• **"Zuppa Toscana" means soup in the style of Tuscany, and I fell in love with it, particularly in the style of Olive Garden. Rich and creamy, this dairy-free version of the classic will take you straight to Italy.**

1 pound Italian-flavored chicken sausage, sliced into disks

1 large onion, diced

2 large turnips, peeled and diced

1 (15-ounce) can cannellini beans, rinsed and drained

1 teaspoon sea salt

½ teaspoon black pepper

¼ teaspoon red pepper flakes

3 garlic cloves, minced

3 cups chicken broth, homemade (page 220) or store-bought

2 teaspoons arrowroot powder

1 cup full-fat coconut milk

6 slices turkey bacon, cooked and crumbled

2 cups (packed) chopped kale

1. Preheat the pressure cooker using the SAUTE function. When the display panel reads HOT, add the sausage and onion, and sauté until the sausage browns and the onion turns translucent, about 5 minutes.

2. Add the turnips, beans, salt, pepper, red pepper flakes, garlic, broth, and arrowroot.

3. Place the lid on the cooker and make sure the pressure knob is in the SEALING position. Using the display panel, press the CANCEL button, then select the MANUAL/PRESSURE COOK function, high pressure, and use the +/- buttons until the display reads 8 minutes.

4. When the cooker beeps to let you know it's finished, switch the pressure knob from the SEALING to the VENTING position, administering a quick release. Use caution while the steam escapes—it's hot.

5. Open the cooker and whisk in the coconut milk, then stir in the turkey bacon and kale. Serve.

*spicy
tomato basil
soup,* PAGE 82

*traditional black bean
soup,* PAGE 86

cleaner corn chowder, PAGE 87

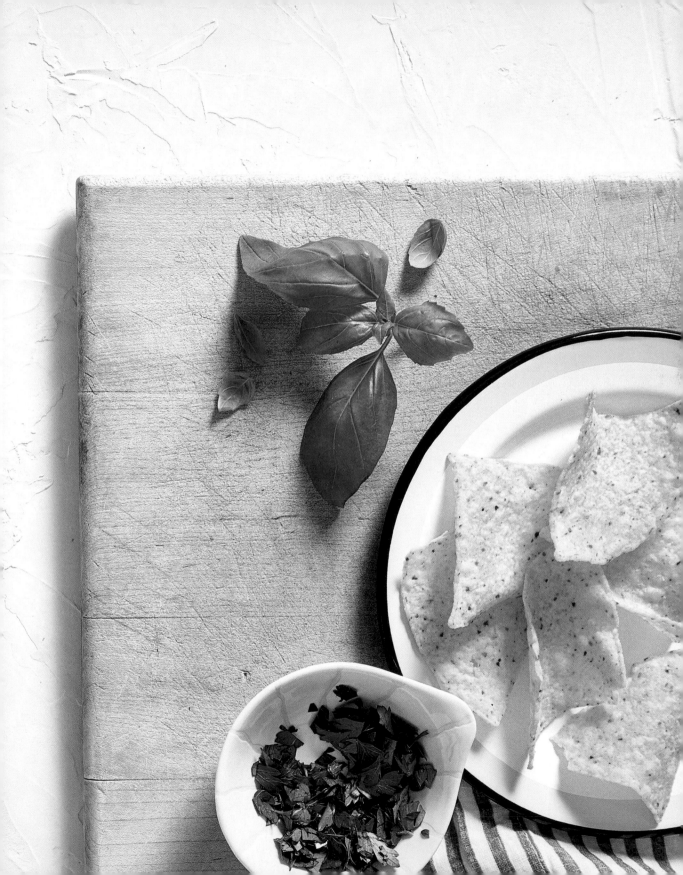

traditional black bean soup

4 cups cooked black beans, homemade (page 226) or canned (2¹/₃ 15-ounce cans), rinsed and drained

2 cups chicken broth, homemade (page 220) or store-bought

½ medium onion, diced

1 tablespoon ground cumin

1 teaspoon sea salt

¼ teaspoon cayenne

¼ cup chopped fresh cilantro

serves 6 • **You'd be surprised at just how fabulous this simple black bean soup tastes. It's very mild, warm, and comforting. It's a perfect side when you're throwing a themed party or it's great as a solo dish any night of the week.**

1. Place all the ingredients, except the cilantro, in a pressure cooker.

2. Put the lid on the cooker and make sure the pressure knob is in the SEALING position. Using the display panel, select the MANUAL/PRESSURE COOK function, high pressure, and use the +/- buttons until the display reads 1 minute.

3. When the cooker beeps to let you know it's finished, switch the pressure knob from the SEALING to the VENTING position, administering a quick release. Use caution while the steam escapes—it's hot.

4. Add the cilantro and serve.

cleaner corn chowder

¼ cup extra-virgin olive oil

4 tablespoons arrowroot powder

1 large onion, diced

2 cups diced celery (about 4 stalks)

2½ cups chicken broth, homemade (page 220) or store-bought

2 cups cubed sweet potatoes (1 to 2 medium)

2½ cups frozen corn kernels

2 teaspoons sea salt

Dash of black pepper

3 garlic cloves, minced

¼ teaspoon red pepper flakes

1 cup Homemade Almond Milk (page 223) or store-bought

serves 6 • **My favorite soup in the entire world is Mimi's Cafe Corn Chowder. I worked there as a teenager and had it for lunch every day for almost a year. It's one of those things I don't ever tire of. After I got married, I found a recipe for it online and it joined our winter dinner rotation. Cutting the dairy out of our diet rendered my traditional recipe useless, so I began trying to make a cleaner version of my old favorite. This chowder is delicious in its own right and definitely hits the spot!**

1. Preheat a pressure cooker using the SAUTE function. When the cooker display panel reads HOT, add the oil and arrowroot powder, whisking to combine.

2. Add the onion and celery, and sauté until the vegetables begin to soften, about 5 minutes. Add the broth, sweet potatoes, corn, salt, pepper, garlic, and red pepper flakes. Stir.

3. Using the display panel, press the CANCEL button, then select the MANUAL/PRESSURE COOK function, high pressure, and use the +/- buttons until the display reads 8 minutes.

4. When the cooker beeps to let you know it's finished, switch the pressure knob from the SEALING to the VENTING position, administering a quick release. Use caution while the steam escapes—it's hot.

5. Open the cooker and add the almond milk. Use an immersion blender and pulse until the soup reaches your preferred consistency.

6. Let cool and serve later; this soup gets better the longer it sits. And it's terrific reheated.

spinach-loaded *veggie soup*

serves 4 to 6 • Who doesn't love a hearty vegetable soup? With plenty of protein from pinto beans, this soup makes a fabulous dinner dish, with no side required. If you're out of spinach and have a bunch of kale on hand, substitute that. Or throw in both kale and spinach for an extra-healthy meal!

1¼ cups dried pinto beans

1 tablespoon extra-virgin olive oil

½ cup diced carrots (2–3 small)

½ cup diced celery (about 1 stalk)

1 medium onion, diced

4 garlic cloves, minced

4 cups vegetable broth, homemade (page 221) or store-bought

1 (15-ounce) can organic diced tomatoes

1½ teaspoons garlic powder

1 teaspoon dried basil

1 teaspoon dried oregano

1 teaspoon sea salt

Dash of black pepper

4 cups baby spinach

1. Cover the pinto beans with water and soak overnight or for 8 hours at room temperature. Rinse and drain.

2. Preheat the pressure cooker using the SAUTE function. When the display panel reads HOT, add the olive oil, carrots, celery, and onion and sauté until the vegetables begin to soften, about 3 minutes.

3. Add the garlic, vegetable broth, tomatoes, garlic powder, basil, oregano, salt, and pepper.

4. Place the lid on the cooker and make sure the pressure knob is in the SEALING position. Using the display panel, press the CANCEL button, then select the SOUP function, high pressure, and use the +/- buttons until the display reads 25 minutes.

5. When the cooker beeps to let you know it's finished, switch the pressure knob from the SEALING to the VENTING position, administering a quick release. Use caution while the steam escapes—it's hot.

6. Open the cooker and stir in the spinach. Serve.

4-minute creamy garlic cauliflower soup

2 tablespoons extra-virgin olive oil

6 slices turkey bacon

5 garlic cloves

1 medium onion, diced

2¹/₂ cups chicken or vegetable broth, homemade (pages 220–21) or store-bought

4 cups chopped cauliflower florets (about 1 head)

¹/₂ teaspoon dried thyme

¹/₂ teaspoon dried rosemary

1 dried bay leaf

Green onions, chopped

Sea salt, to taste

serves 4 to 6 • **This light and flavorful soup comes together in a flash and is great accompanied by a Simple Chicken Caesar Salad (page 100) or Grain-Free Garlic Biscuits (page 185).**

1. Preheat a pressure cooker using the SAUTE function. When the display panel reads HOT, add the oil and bacon, and sauté until crisp. Remove the bacon and set aside. Add the garlic and onion, and sauté until softened and translucent, about 5 minutes.

2. Deglaze the cooker with a bit of the broth, stirring up all the browned bits. Add the cauliflower, thyme, rosemary, remaining broth, and the bay leaf.

3. Place the lid on the cooker and make sure the pressure knob is in the SEALING position. Using the display panel, press the CANCEL button, then select the SOUP function, high pressure, and use the +/- buttons until the display reads 4 minutes.

4. When the cooker beeps to let you know it's finished, switch the pressure knob from the SEALING to the VENTING position, administering a quick release. Use caution while the steam escapes—it's hot.

5. Open the cooker and remove the bay leaf. Use an immersion blender to puree the soup. Garnish with the green onions and crumbled turkey bacon and season with salt.

chicken tortilla *soup*

serves 6 • **When I first started posting recipes online, I would constantly get requests for a chicken tortilla soup. I designed this recipe with my readers in my mind, and to this day it remains one of my most popular recipes. Add a little avocado, guacamole, sour cream, cheese—whatever your heart desires. This one is a winner.**

2 (6- to 8-ounce) frozen boneless, skinless chicken breasts

2 cups cooked black beans, homemade (page 226) or canned, rinsed and drained

2 cups frozen corn kernels

5 garlic cloves

1 large onion, diced

1 red bell pepper, diced

6 ounces organic tomato paste

4 cups chicken or vegetable broth, homemade (pages 220–21) or store-bought

1/2 cup diced pickled jalapeños, with juice

1/4 cup taco seasoning, preferably homemade (page 231)

Diced avocado, tortilla strips, and chopped fresh cilantro, for garnish

1. Place all the ingredients in a pressure cooker except for the garnishes.

2. Put the lid on the cooker and make sure the pressure knob is in the SEALING position. Using the display panel, select the MANUAL function, high pressure, and use the +/- buttons until the display reads 15 minutes.

3. When the cooker beeps to let you know it's finished, switch the pressure knob from the SEALING to the VENTING position, administering a quick release. Use caution while the steam escapes—it's hot.

4. Remove the lid and shred the chicken. Combine with the remaining cooked ingredients and serve, topped with the avocado, tortilla strips, and cilantro.

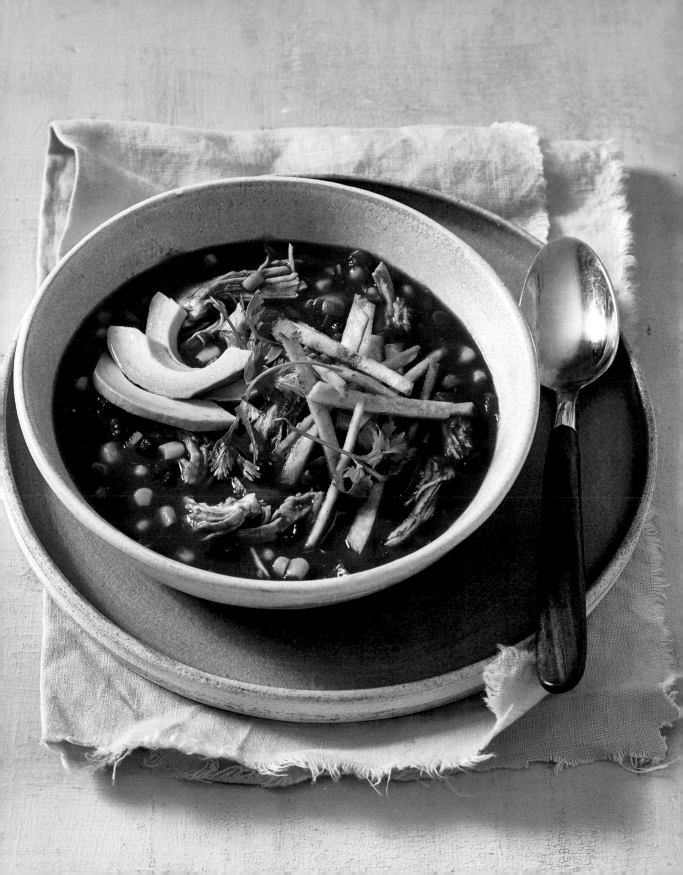

fire-roasted beef stew

serves 8 • **If you ask my husband what he wants to eat, 99 times out of 100 he requests a beef dish. I have several different beef stew recipes but this is his all-time favorite.**

2 pounds cubed beef stew meat

1 large onion, diced

1 (15-ounce) can organic fire-roasted tomatoes, diced

1 cup beef or chicken broth, homemade (page 220) or store-bought

¼ cup dried minced onion

¼ cup dried parsley

1 tablespoon chili powder

1 teaspoon black pepper

3 cups baby carrots

3 cups cubed sweet potatoes (1 to 2 medium)

2 cups chopped celery (about 4 stalks)

2 cups sliced white button mushrooms

5 garlic cloves, chopped or thinly sliced

1 tablespoon extra-virgin olive oil

½ tablespoon ghee (optional)

2 teaspoons sea salt, plus more to taste

1. Put the beef, onion, tomatoes, broth, minced onion, parsley, chili powder, and pepper in a pressure cooker.

2. Place the lid on the cooker and make sure the pressure knob is in the SEALING position. Using the display panel, select the MANUAL function, high pressure, and use the +/- buttons until the display reads 40 minutes. If your meat is frozen, as mine normally is, add an extra 20 minutes (display at 60).

3. When the cooker beeps to let you know it's finished, switch the pressure knob from the SEALING to the VENTING position, administering a quick release. Use caution while the steam escapes—it's hot.

4. Add the carrots, sweet potatoes, celery, mushrooms, garlic, olive oil, ghee (if using), and salt.

5. Place the lid back on the cooker and make sure the pressure knob is in the SEALING position. Using the display panel, select the MANUAL function, high pressure, and use the +/- buttons until the display reads 10 minutes.

6. When the cooker beeps to let you know it's finished, switch the pressure knob from the SEALING to the VENTING position, administering a quick release. Use caution while the steam escapes—it's hot.

7. Open the cooker and stir everything in the pot; adjust salt to taste.

super-simple *chili*

1½ cups dried pinto beans

1 pound lean ground beef

1 tablespoon dried minced onion

1½ tablespoons garlic powder

¼ teaspoon sea salt

⅛ teaspoon black pepper

3 (15-ounce) cans organic tomato sauce

3 tablespoons chili powder

serves 6 • **Trust me, you're not going to find a chili with a shorter ingredient list or easier prep. And this chili tastes great, too. You can swap the dried beans for two cans of rinsed and drained; just make sure you cut the cooking time to ten minutes.**

1. Soak the beans overnight in water to cover, then rinse and drain.

2. Preheat the pressure cooker using the SAUTE function. When the display panel reads HOT, add the ground beef along with the onion, garlic powder, salt, and pepper. Cook until the meat is browned, about 10 minutes.

3. Press the CANCEL button and add the beans, tomato sauce, and chili powder. **Do not stir.**

4. Put the lid on the cooker and make sure the vent valve is in the SEALING position. Using the display panel, press the CANCEL button, then select the BEAN/CHILI button. If your cooker does not have this button, select the MANUAL/ PRESSURE COOK function, high pressure, and use the +/- until the display reads 30 minutes.

5. When the cooker beeps to let you know it's finished, switch the pressure knob from the SEALING to the VENTING position, administering a quick release. Use caution while the steam escapes—it's hot.

6. Open the cooker and serve.

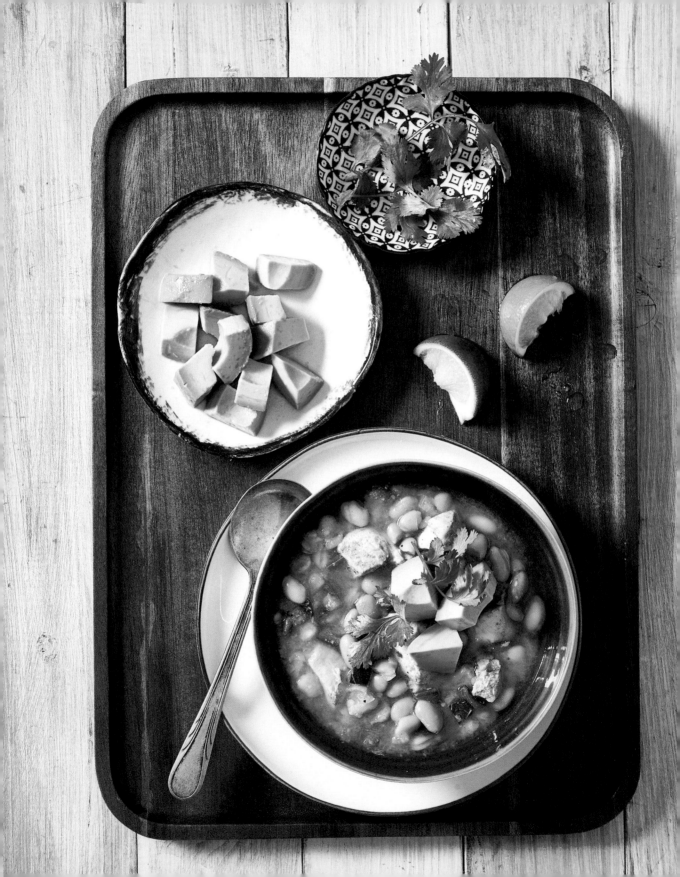

5-minute poblano chicken chili

½ tablespoon extra-virgin olive oil

1 teaspoon ground cumin

1 teaspoon dried minced onion

1 teaspoon sea salt

½ teaspoon garlic powder

¼ teaspoon cayenne

¼ teaspoon black pepper

1 medium onion, diced

2 poblano chiles, ribbed and seeded

1 jalapeño, diced (ribbed and seeded if you don't like it spicy)

1 (8-ounce) boneless, skinless chicken breast, cubed

2 (15-ounce) cans great northern beans, rinsed and drained

1½ cups chicken broth, homemade (page 220) or store-bought

½ cup chopped fresh cilantro

Lemon or lime quarters

Diced avocado (optional)

serves 4 to 6 • **This white chicken chili is full of flavor and spice. High in protein and fiber, it's very filling and will keep you feeling satisfied until your next meal!**

1. Preheat a pressure cooker using the SAUTE function. When the display panel reads HOT, add the oil, cumin, minced onion, salt, garlic powder, cayenne, black pepper, onion, poblanos, jalapeño, and chicken. Sauté until the chicken begins to turn white and the onion becomes translucent, about 5 minutes.

2. Add the beans and broth.

3. Place the lid on the cooker and make sure the pressure knob is in the SEALING position. Using the display panel, select the MANUAL/PRESSURE COOK function, high pressure, and use the +/- buttons until the display reads 5 minutes.

4. When the cooker beeps to let you know it's finished, switch the pressure knob from the SEALING to the VENTING position, administering a quick release. Use caution while the steam escapes—it's hot.

5. Open the cooker and stir in the cilantro. Squeeze some lemon or lime juice over and top with avocado, if using.

SALADS
and
WRAPS

cobb *salad*

2 (8-ounce) boneless, skinless chicken breasts, grilled or baked

1 head of romaine lettuce, chopped

2 cups baby spinach

1/2 cup shredded red cabbage

2 hard-boiled eggs, diced (see page 187)

1 avocado, diced

1 Roma (plum) tomato, diced

6 slices turkey bacon, cooked and crumbled

Homemade Ranch Dressing (recipe follows)

serves 4 to 6 • I have always been a fan of big leafy green salads, even as a kid. Salad is a BIG part of our diet. It was important for me to get my kids eating salad early on so that it would be something they *wanted* to eat. And there's something else I love about salads: You can turn almost anything into one! This salad is reminiscent of a hearty chicken-bacon club sandwich.

1. Cut the chicken into thin strips.

2. Place the romaine, spinach, and cabbage in a large bowl. Toss well.

3. Top with the eggs, avocado, and tomato, then add the chicken and the bacon.

4. Drizzle with the dressing and serve.

homemade ranch dressing

makes 2 cups • My Aunt Kim turned our family onto homemade ranch dressing. My husband was a HUGE Hidden Valley fan, but we created our own version free of MSG, high-fructose corn syrup, and preservatives. This dressing will knock your socks off. It's great on a salad, as a veggie dip, or mixed with my Homemade Barbecue Sauce (page 130).

3/4 cup Homemade Mayonnaise (page 224) or store-bought

1/2 cup sour cream, Greek, or coconut yogurt

1 tablespoon water

1 teaspoon dried minced onion

1 teaspoon dried parsley

1/2 teaspoon garlic powder

Place all the ingredients in a high-powered blender. Blend until smooth.

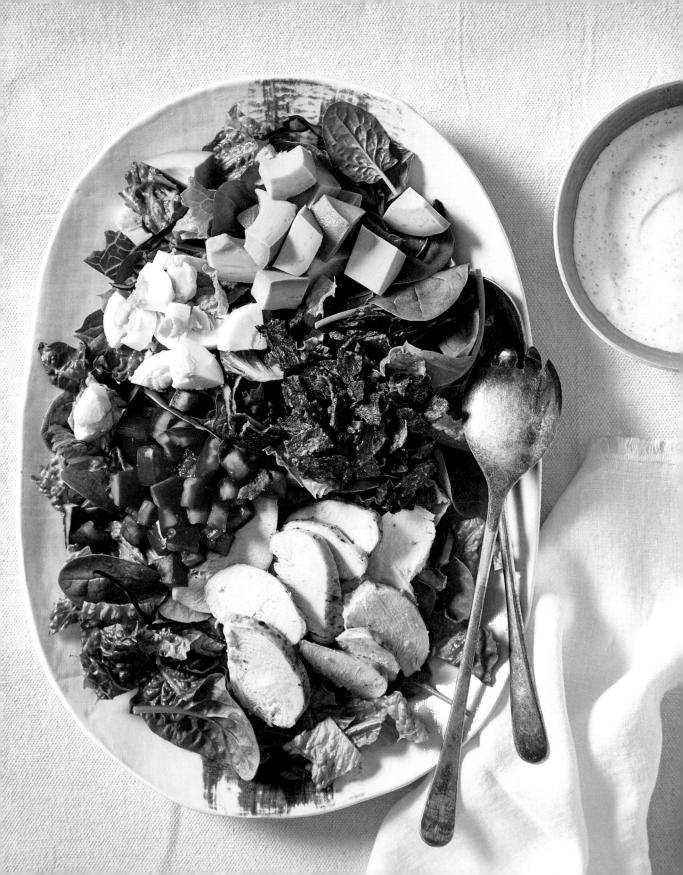

simple chicken caesar salad

1 pound boneless, skinless chicken breast

1 tablespoon extra-virgin olive oil

1 teaspoon sea salt

1/4 teaspoon black pepper

1 head of romaine lettuce, chopped

4 cups chopped baby spinach

1/3 cup raw cashews, grated

1 recipe Simple Caesar Dressing (recipe follows)

serves 4 • One of my biggest inspirations is cooking healthier versions of my loved ones' favorite foods. My sister Bethany loves chicken Caesar salad, so I wanted to create a special recipe just for her! Now we eat it even when she's not around.

1. Preheat the oven to 375°F.

2. Place the chicken in a bowl. Drizzle with the olive oil and sprinkle with the salt and pepper. Toss until coated.

3. Place the chicken in a roasting pan or baking dish and bake for 35 to 40 minutes, depending on thickness.

4. Remove the chicken from the oven and let rest for 10 minutes. Cut into bite-size pieces and serve over the romaine and spinach. Sprinkle with the cashews and drizzle with the dressing.

simple caesar dressing

makes 1/2 cup • This dressing is sans the anchovies because who keeps anchovies on hand, anyway?

1/4 cup Homemade Mayonnaise (page 224) or store-bought

2 tablespoons avocado oil

1/2 teaspoon low-sodium Worcestershire sauce

1/4 teaspoon organic Dijon mustard

Pinch of black pepper

Sea salt

Place all the ingredients in a wide-mouth mason jar and pulse with an immersion blender until combined. (Alternatively, you can use a blender and process until smooth.) Adjust salt to taste.

strawberry, spinach, and pecan *salad*

4 cups chopped baby spinach

2 cups sliced fresh strawberries

¼ cup pecans, chopped

⅓ cup avocado oil

1 tablespoon pure maple syrup

1 tablespoon dried minced onion

¼ teaspoon low-sodium Worcestershire sauce

2 tablespoons sesame seeds

1 teaspoon chia seeds

serves 4 • I love big, hearty salads, but there is also something nice about a light, dainty salad, especially this one with its gorgeous colors and fresh flavors. There's a feminine quality to this salad, so it's great for bridal showers, baby showers, and potlucks. It's light enough to be a side, but it can satisfy as a main course, as well.

1. Combine the spinach, strawberries, and pecans in a large bowl. Toss to combine.

2. Whisk together the oil, maple syrup, onion, Worcestershire sauce, sesame seeds, and chia seeds to form a dressing.

3. Drizzle the dressing on the salad and serve.

*summer
asparagus-
squash salad,*
PAGE 103

*strawberry,
spinach, and pecan
salad,* PAGE 101

summer asparagus-squash salad

1 medium zucchini, cut into bite-size pieces

1 medium yellow squash, cut into bite-size pieces

10 asparagus, cut into bite-size pieces

1 jalapeño, cut into bite-size pieces

3 tablespoons Homemade Mayonnaise (page 224) or store-bought

½ to 1 teaspoon red wine vinegar

½ teaspoon sea salt

¼ teaspoon black pepper

¼ teaspoon garlic powder

serves 4 • **Need a side to bring to a potluck? Look no further! This simple little salad is a refreshing bite at a summer gathering, or any other time of year if you like! It's easy to throw together and a great way to get your veggies. The longer this stays chilled before serving, the better it is!**

1. Pour 1 cup water into a pressure cooker. Set a vegetable steamer basket inside the cooker.

2. Place the zucchini, squash, and asparagus in the basket.

3. Put the lid on the cooker and make sure the pressure knob is in the SEALING position. Using the display panel, select the STEAM function, low pressure, and use the +/- buttons until the display reads 0.

4. When the cooker beeps to let you know it's finished, switch the pressure knob from the SEALING to the VENTING position, administering a quick release. Use caution while the steam escapes—it's hot.

5. Open the cooker and immediately remove the veggies (leaving them in the pot will cause them to overcook) and place in the refrigerator to chill for 3 hours or overnight.

6. When ready to serve, place the chilled veggies in a large bowl and add the jalapeño, mayo, and vinegar (start with ½ teaspoon and increase to 1 teaspoon for a more acidic kick!), and season with the salt, pepper, and garlic powder. Stir until combined. Serve chilled. (Salad can be stored in the refrigerator until serving time.)

tuna salad *with* plantains

My husband, Brady, is a no-frills guy. He's an engineer, very matter of fact. When we were first dating, he invited me over and made me tuna fish salad served with Ritz crackers for dinner! I loved how no-nonsense that was. While we don't eat those crackers anymore, we do still make a great tuna salad. This dish takes me back to that very first, simple dinner.

2 (5-ounce) cans wild-caught tuna, drained

⅓ cup Homemade Mayonnaise (page 224) or store-bought

⅓ cup sweet relish

¼ cup diced orange or yellow bell pepper

1 head of romaine lettuce, leaves separated

1 cup shredded red cabbage

8 ounces plantain chips, crushed

1. Place the tuna in a bowl and mix in the mayonnaise, relish, and bell pepper.

2. Fill each romaine leaf with a healthy scoop of tuna salad and top with a sprinkling of cabbage and plantain crumbs.

sweet and savory lightened-up chicken salad

2 (8-ounce) boneless, skinless chicken breasts

Sea salt

Black pepper

3/4 cup Homemade Mayonnaise (page 224) or store-bought

1 cup diced celery (about 2 stalks)

1 cup purple grapes, halved and quartered

1/2 cup pecans, chopped

2 teaspoons dried dillweed

1 head of butterleaf lettuce, leaves separated (optional)

serves 4 • **The dill really gives this salad a bright, fresh flavor that I can't get enough of. This salad remains a staple in my kitchen, and I hope it finds a home in yours as well.**

1. Lightly season the chicken with salt and pepper.

2. Add 1 cup water to a pressure cooker. Put the trivet in the cooker and then place the chicken breasts on the trivet.

3. Put the lid on the cooker and make sure the vent valve is in the SEALING position. Using the display panel, select the POULTRY button, high pressure, for 6 minutes. (If your cooker does not have this function, select the MANUAL/PRESSURE COOK function, high pressure, for 6 minutes.)

4. When the cooker beeps to let you know it's finished, let it naturally come down from pressure until the display reads LO:15. This will keep your chicken tender. Switch the vent valve from the SEALING to the VENTING position. Use caution while the steam escapes—it's hot.

5. Transfer the chicken to a large bowl and use a fork to shred it.

6. Add the mayo, celery, grapes, pecans, dill, and 1/4 to 1/2 teaspoon salt. Stir well. Serve as is or use the lettuce leaves to make wraps.

asian chicken *lettuce* *wraps*

2 (8-ounce) boneless, skinless chicken breasts

Sea salt

1 teaspoon garlic powder

2 tablespoons extra-virgin olive oil

1/4 cup chopped fresh cilantro

1/4 cup avocado oil

1 garlic clove, finely chopped

1 1/2 tablespoons agave nectar

1 head of butterleaf or Bibb lettuce, leaves separated

1/2 cup shredded carrots (about 2 medium)

1/2 cup matchstick-cut cucumber

1/2 cup shredded red cabbage

1 cup bean sprouts

1/3 cup raw cashews, grated

serves 4 • **My absolute favorite restaurant is the Cheesecake Factory. They have a neat little Skinnylicious menu that caters to special diets, and my favorite on that menu is the Asian Chicken Lettuce Wraps. Technically an appetizer, these wraps are also satisfying as a main course. When we stopped eating out, I dedicated myself to re-creating my favorite restaurant recipes so that I could enjoy them at home. These wraps are full of flavor and all kinds of yummy. Suggestion: use a food processor to grate the cashews.**

1. Heat a skillet over medium heat. Meanwhile, season the chicken breasts with 1 teaspoon salt and the garlic powder.

2. Add the olive oil to the skillet and then add the chicken. Adjust the heat to medium-low and cook for about 5 minutes, until white and firm.

3. Process the cilantro, avocado oil, garlic, agave, and a pinch of salt in a blender until smooth (or use an immersion blender). Set the dressing aside.

4. Turn the chicken over, and cook on the other side until cooked through, about 8 minutes more.

5. Let the chicken cool somewhat to set the juices, then cut into thin slices.

6. Place the carrots, cucumber, cabbage, sprouts, and cashews in separate bowls for easy assembly.

7. Drizzle the chicken slices with the cilantro dressing and serve with the lettuce leaves and ingredients for self-assembly of the wraps, as desired.

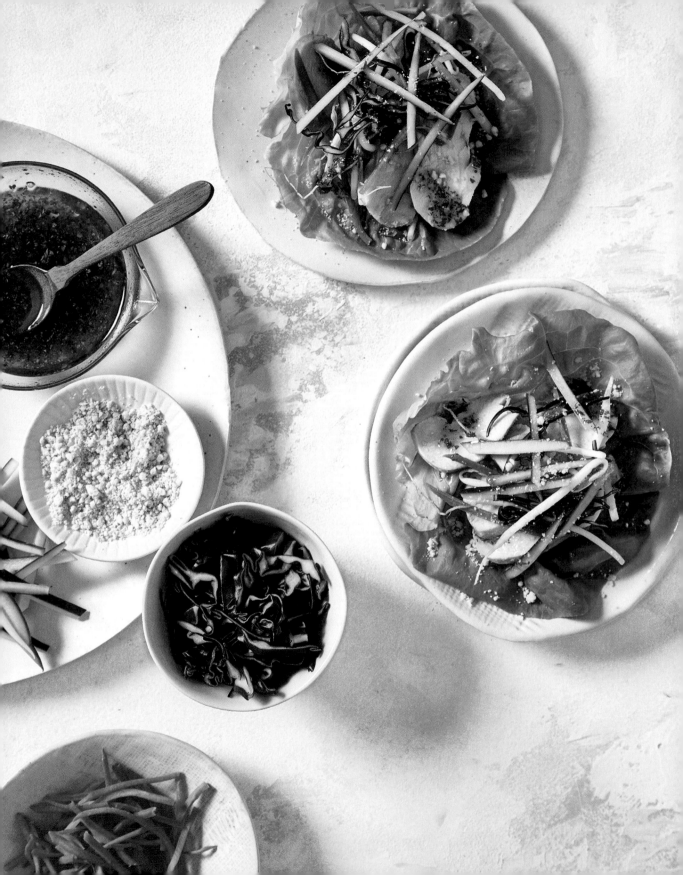

egg salad *lettuce wraps*

8 eggs

2 tablespoons organic mustard

3 tablespoons Homemade Mayonnaise (page 224) or store-bought

½ cup diced dill pickles

½ teaspoon apple cider vinegar

¼ teaspoon dried minced onion

¼ teaspoon sea salt

⅛ teaspoon black pepper

¼ teaspoon paprika

1 head of butterleaf or romaine lettuce, leaves separated

1 cup broccoli slaw

1 ripe medium tomato, diced

serves 4 • **My son loves hard-boiled eggs—he could easily eat five of them in one sitting—so all shortcuts are welcomed. Here's an alternative way to prepare hard-boiled eggs in your pressure cooker if you don't want to peel the shells off the cooked eggs. You crack the eggs straight into a baking dish that fits inside the pressure cooker, cover with foil, and cook. Voilà! You have an egg loaf! Just chop it up—no peeling required.**

1. Place 1 cup water in a pressure cooker. Put the trivet or a steamer basket inside and stack the eggs in it.

2. Put the lid on the cooker and make sure the vent valve is in the SEALING position. Using the display panel, select the MANUAL/PRESSURE COOK function, high pressure, and use the +/- buttons until the display reads 5 minutes.

3. When the cooker beeps to let you know it's finished, let it naturally come down from pressure until the display reads LO:, switch the vent valve from the SEALING to the VENTING position. Use caution while the steam escapes—it's hot. Do not let it naturally release for any more than 5 minutes or you will overcook your eggs.

4. Open the cooker and immediately plunge the eggs into an ice bath to halt the cooking process.

5. Peel and dice the eggs.

6. In a bowl, combine the eggs with the mustard, mayo, pickles, vinegar, onion, salt, pepper, and paprika.

7. Spread each lettuce leaf with some egg salad, broccoli slaw, and tomato. Wrap and enjoy!

honey mustard–turkey bacon *wrap*

serves 4 • **In our house, we're gluten free, so instead of making sandwiches, we make wrapwiches. You'll be surprised how satisfying a lettuce wrap can be with the proper fillings and condiments!**

8 ounces cooked turkey breast, thinly sliced

1 head of butterleaf or leaf lettuce

6 slices turkey bacon, cooked until crisp and diced

2 Roma (plum) tomatoes, diced

½ avocado, diced

½ cup chopped fresh parsley

½ cup thinly sliced green onions

Honey Mustard Dressing (recipe follows)

Assemble the wraps by placing one or two slices of turkey in a leaf, then top with the turkey bacon, tomatoes, and avocado. Finish with a sprinkling of parsley and green onion. Drizzle on the dressing and wrap.

honey mustard dressing

makes 1 cup • **My dad used to order a side salad with honey mustard dressing every time we went out to eat when I was a kid. I have fond memories of picking out the croutons on his plate, doused with the dressing. This is a cleaner version of this comforting favorite. It's also dynamite as a dip with my Turkey Nuggets (page 147)!**

½ cup Homemade Mayonnaise (page 224) or store-bought

1 tablespoon organic yellow mustard

1 tablespoon low-sodium Worcestershire sauce

½ teaspoon organic raw honey

Place all the ingredients in a wide-mouth mason jar and pulse with an immersion blender until combined. (Or combine in a blender.) (The dressing will keep in the fridge for 10 to 14 days.)

QUICK
AND EASY
ONE-BOWL
MEALS

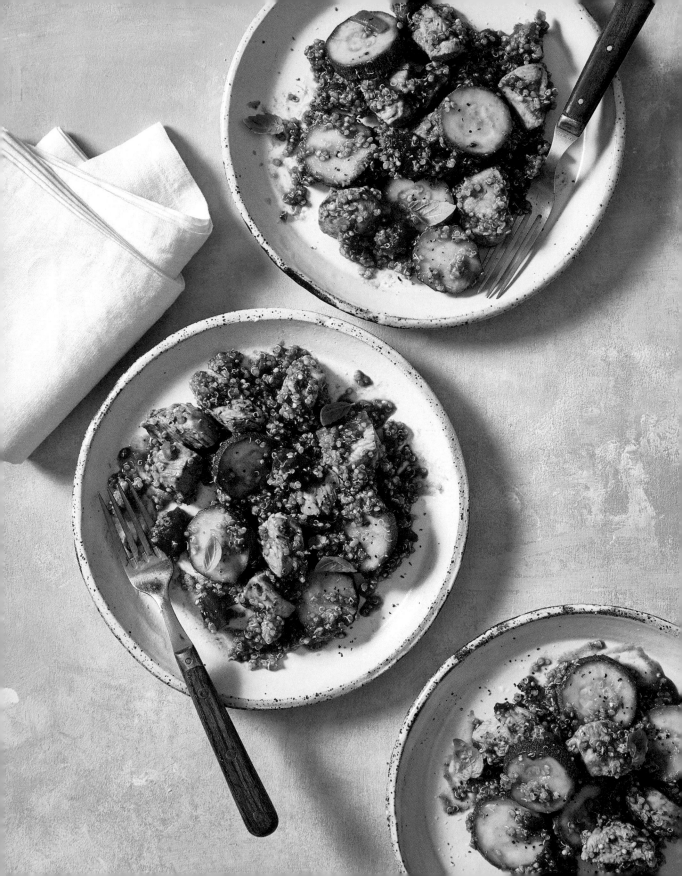

zucchine basilico *bowl*

2 tablespoons extra-virgin olive oil

1 medium red onion, diced

2 garlic cloves, finely chopped

1½ pounds boneless, skinless chicken breast, bite-size pieces

1 teaspoon sea salt

½ teaspoon black pepper

1 cup quinoa, rinsed and drained

2 (14.5-ounce) cans organic diced tomatoes

1 teaspoon red pepper flakes

½ cup fresh basil, minced, or 1 tablespoon dried Italian seasoning

½ tablespoon garlic powder

1 dried bay leaf

2 pounds or 3 small unpeeled zucchini, cut in ½-inch slices

serves 6 • **Inspired by authentic Italian cuisine, this is one of my family's favorite dishes. The fresh basil really makes the dish sing!**

1. Preheat a pressure cooker using the SAUTE function. When the display panel reads HOT, add the olive oil and onion. Sauté until the onion begins to soften, about 5 minutes.

2. Add the garlic, chicken, 1 teaspoon of the salt, and ½ teaspoon of the pepper. Let the chicken cook for 5 minutes on one side, then turn it over and cook for 3 more minutes.

3. Add the quinoa, tomatoes, red pepper flakes, basil, garlic powder, bay leaf, and zucchini. **Do not stir.**

4. Place the lid on the cooker and make sure the pressure knob is in the SEALING position. Using the display panel, select the MANUAL/PRESSURE COOK function, high pressure, and use the +/- buttons until the display reads 1 minute.

5. When the cooker beeps to let you know it's finished, let it naturally come down from pressure until the display reads LO:25. Switch the pressure knob from the SEALING to the VENTING position. Use caution while the steam escapes—it's hot.

6. Open the cooker and remove the bay leaf. Stir, and serve.

light and fresh *mediterranean bowl*

½ cup quinoa, rinsed and drained

1 cup chicken broth, homemade (page 220) or store-bought; or water

¼ teaspoon garlic powder

¼ teaspoon dried minced onion

¼ teaspoon sea salt

½ cup diced red bell pepper

¼ cup pitted Kalamata olives, diced

1 tablespoon chopped fresh parsley

3 tablespoons chopped green onions

¼ cup fresh lemon juice

1 teaspoon balsamic vinegar

1 tablespoon olive oil

serves 2 • **With the right blend of vegetables, herbs, and spices, this fresh Mediterranean dish is the perfect balance of delicious and light. And since making quinoa in a pressure cooker is even quicker than on the stovetop, this meal can be made in under 20 minutes.**

1. Place the quinoa in a pressure cooker. Add the broth, garlic powder, onion, and salt.

2. Place the lid on the cooker and make sure the pressure knob is in the SEALING position. Using the display panel, select the MANUAL/PRESSURE COOK function, high pressure, and use the +/- buttons until the display reads 1 minute.

3. When the cooker beeps to let you know it's finished, let it naturally come down from pressure until the display reads LO:10. Switch the pressure knob from the SEALING to the VENTING position. Use caution while the steam escapes—it's hot.

4. Transfer the quinoa to a serving bowl and fluff with a fork. (Transferring it will stop the cooking process and prevent it from becoming mushy.) Add the bell pepper, olives, parsley, green onion, lemon juice, vinegar, and olive oil. Stir to combine, and serve.

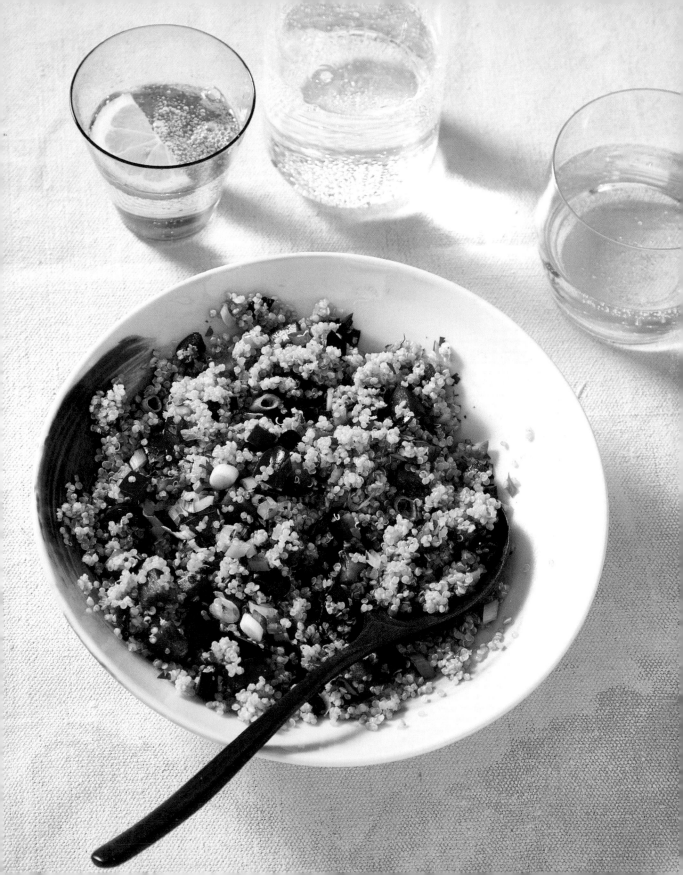

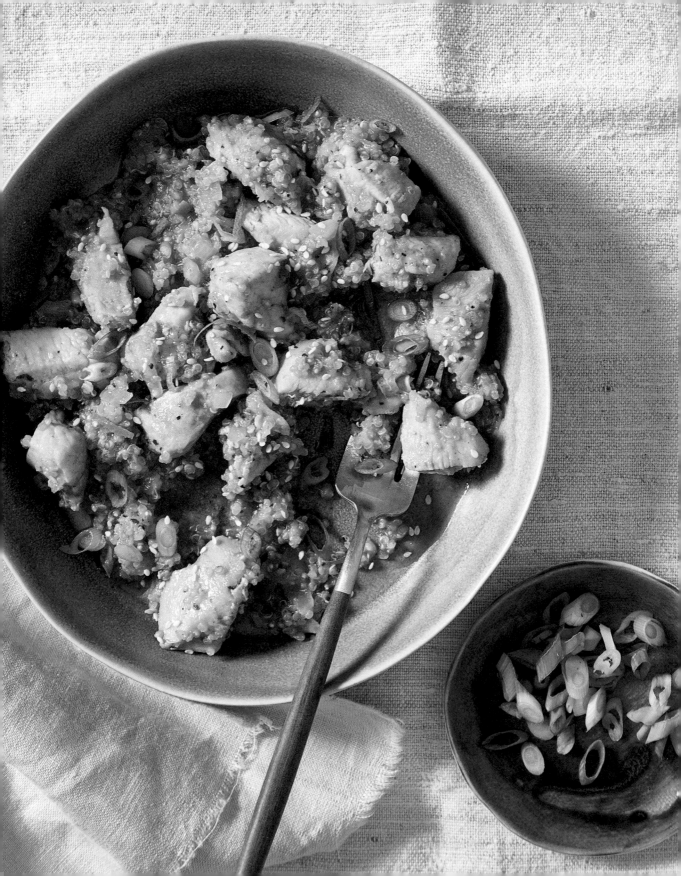

better than takeout orange chicken bowl

2 tablespoons avocado oil

1 pound boneless, skinless chicken breast, cut into bite-size pieces

1 small onion, diced

1 teaspoon sea salt

½ teaspoon black pepper

¼ teaspoon red pepper flakes

½ cup quinoa, rinsed and drained

½ cup chicken broth, homemade (page 220) or store-bought

Orange Ginger Dressing (recipe follows)

¼ cup chopped green onions (optional)

1 tablespoon sesame seeds (optional)

serves 4 • **Forget ordering out! This orange chicken will have you breaking up with your takeout joint in favor of a much more flavorful and healthier alternative!**

1. Preheat a pressure cooker using the SAUTE function. When the display panel reads HOT, add the oil, chicken, onion, salt, black pepper, and red pepper flakes.

2. Cook the chicken on one side for 5 minutes, then turn it over and cook for 3 more minutes.

3. Add the quinoa and broth, and stir.

4. Place the lid on the cooker and make sure the pressure knob is in the SEALING position. Using the display panel, select the MANUAL/ PRESSURE COOK function, high pressure, and use the +/- buttons until the display reads 1 minute.

5. When the cooker beeps to let you know it's finished, let it naturally come down from pressure until the display reads LO:6. Switch the pressure knob from the SEALING to the VENTING position. Use caution while the steam escapes—it's hot.

6. Add ½ cup of the dressing to the pot. Stir to incorporate, and serve warm, sprinkled with the green onion and sesame seeds, if using.

recipe continues

orange ginger dressing

makes 1 cup • **Deliciously tangy, this dressing is delightful over a fresh Chinese chicken salad, too.**

2 garlic cloves, finely chopped

1/4 cup organic raw honey

1 teaspoon grated orange zest

1/4 cup fresh orange juice

3 tablespoons coconut aminos

2 tablespoons rice vinegar

2 tablespoons arrowroot powder

1/2 teaspoon grated fresh ginger

1/4 teaspoon black pepper

Place all the ingredients in a high-powered blender and process until smooth.

egg roll bowl

serves 4 • **A Chinese-American classic converted to a bowl dish! This alternative version features the same delicious flavors, but with fresh, whole-foods ingredients and no frying. Take that, takeout!**

1 tablespoon toasted sesame oil

1 (8-ounce) boneless, skinless chicken breast, thinly sliced, around 2 1/2 inches

1 medium onion, diced

1/2 teaspoon sea salt

1/4 teaspoon red pepper flakes

1/2 teaspoon black pepper

1/8 teaspoon grated fresh ginger

2 garlic cloves, finely chopped

1/2 cup quinoa, rinsed and drained

1 cup canned coconut milk

1 cup shredded carrots (about 3 medium)

2 cups shredded red cabbage

1 tablespoon coconut aminos

1 tablespoon rice wine vinegar

1 tablespoon organic raw honey

1. Preheat a pressure cooker using the SAUTE function. When the display panel reads HOT, add the sesame oil, chicken, onion, salt, red pepper flakes, black pepper, ginger, and garlic.

2. Cook the chicken for 5 minutes on one side, then turn it over and cook for 3 more minutes.

3. Add the quinoa, coconut milk, carrots, cabbage, coconut aminos, vinegar, and honey. Stir to combine.

4. Place the lid on the cooker and make sure the pressure knob is in the SEALING position. Using the display panel, select the MANUAL/PRESSURE COOK function, high pressure, and use the +/- buttons until the display reads 1 minute.

5. When the cooker beeps to let you know it's finished, let it naturally come down from pressure until the display reads LO:6. Switch the pressure knob from the SEALING to the VENTING position. Use caution while the steam escapes—it's hot.

6. Open the cooker and serve.

skinny chicken pot pie

1 tablespoon extra-virgin olive oil

2 (8-ounce) boneless, skinless chicken breasts, cut into bite-size pieces

1 medium red onion, diced

½ teaspoon sea salt, plus more to taste

¼ teaspoon black pepper

1 cup chicken broth, homemade (page 220) or store-bought

½ cup quinoa, rinsed and drained

¼ cup full-fat coconut milk

¼ cup coconut aminos

3 tablespoons organic raw honey

1 tablespoon dried parsley

1 teaspoon garlic powder

½ teaspoon ground cumin

3 cups frozen mixed vegetables (peas, corn, carrots, green beans)

serves 6 • **"I don't need the crust!" is what you'll say after trying this skinny version of a pot pie.**

1. Preheat a pressure cooker using the SAUTE function, and press the button until the display panel reads MORE. When the display panel reads HOT, add the oil, chicken, onion, salt, and ⅛ teaspoon of the pepper. Cook the chicken for 5 minutes on one side, then turn the pieces over and cook for 3 more minutes, or until they are browned on all sides and the onion is translucent.

2. Add the broth, quinoa, coconut milk, coconut aminos, honey, parsley, garlic powder, cumin, remaining ⅛ teaspoon pepper, and mixed vegetables. **Do not stir.**

3. Place the lid on the cooker and make sure the pressure knob is in the SEALING position. Using the display panel, press the CANCEL button, then select the MANUAL/PRESSURE COOK function, high pressure, and use the +/- buttons until the display reads 1 minute.

4. When the cooker beeps to let you know it's finished, let it naturally come down from pressure until the display reads LO:10. Switch the pressure knob from the SEALING to the VENTING position. Use caution while the steam escapes—it's hot.

5. Open the cooker and taste. Adjust the seasoning with additional salt, if desired, and serve.

note: This is also a great "dump meal"! Just toss everything into the pot in the order listed, then select the MANUAL function. Cook on high pressure for 10 minutes and let the pot naturally release for 10 minutes!

vegan
fajita bowl

2 red or green bell peppers, seeded and thinly sliced

1 large onion, thinly sliced

1 jalapeño, thinly sliced (seeded, if you don't like it spicy)

Sea salt, to taste

1 head of romaine lettuce, chopped

2 cups chopped baby spinach

1 cup Cilantro Lime Rice (page 191)

2 cups cooked black beans, homemade (page 226) or canned, rinsed and drained

2 Roma (plum) tomatoes, diced

1 avocado, diced

1 cup your favorite sugar-free salsa

serves 4 to 6 • **Who says you need meat to make a delicious fajita? One taste of this bowl and you'll realize a vegan fajita bowl is not only doable but also delicious! Packed with sautéed peppers and onion, fresh spinach, lettuce, and more, this satisfies our family's craving for Mexican cuisine.**

1. Preheat a pressure cooker using the SAUTE function. When the display panel reads HOT, add the bell peppers, onion, jalapeño, and salt. Sauté for 12 to 20 minutes or until the peppers begin to blacken and soften.

2. Assemble the bowls. Place a layer of lettuce and spinach in the bottom of each, then layer in the rice, beans, tomatoes, and avocado. Add the pepper mixture, and top with salsa.

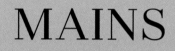

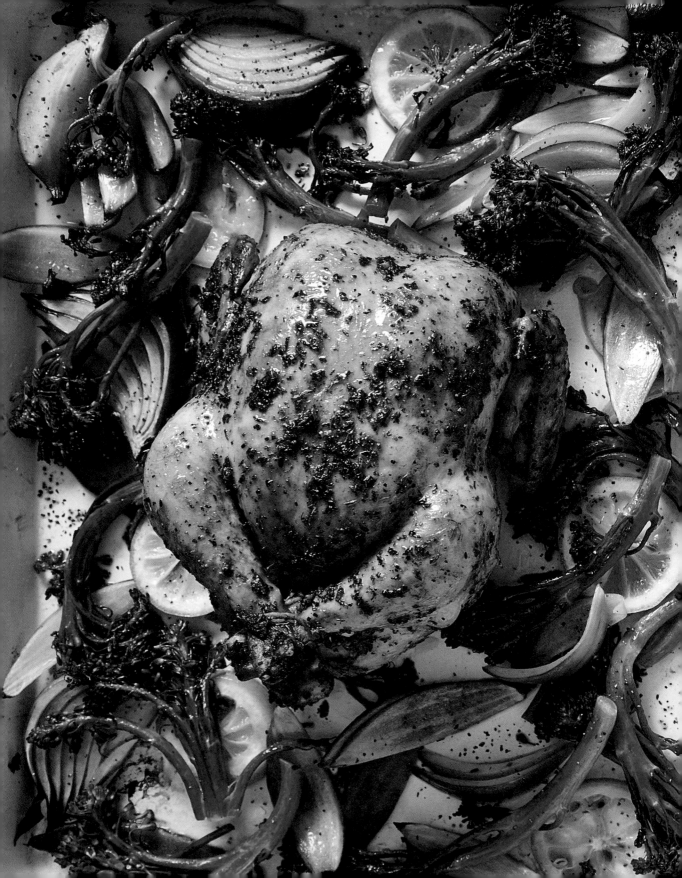

marinated *fall-off-the-bone* herb chicken

1 (3- to 4-pound) chicken

Sea salt, to taste

2 teaspoons dried oregano

2 teaspoons dried parsley

2 teaspoons dried basil

1 teaspoon dried thyme

1 teaspoon dried sage

1 teaspoon black pepper

4 garlic cloves, finely chopped

½ cup extra-virgin olive oil

½ cup water

serves 6 • **The trick to cooking a perfect flavorful chicken in the pressure cooker is to marinate it first. This requires a little bit of planning, but it pays off big time. If your chicken is bigger than 3 to 4 pounds, add 6 minutes of cooking time for each additional pound.**

1. Place the chicken in a medium-large bowl. Liberally rub the chicken with salt, getting it into every crevice, inside and out.

2. Sprinkle the chicken with the oregano, parsley, basil, thyme, sage, pepper, and garlic. Drizzle with the olive oil, making sure the bird is throughly coated. Cover the bowl with plastic wrap and place in the refrigerator for 4 to 8 hours.

3. Add ½ cup water to a pressure cooker. Place the trivet inside and carefully place the chicken on top. Discard any liquid remaining in the bowl.

4. Place the lid on the cooker and make sure the pressure knob is in the SEALING position. Using the display panel, select the MANUAL function, high pressure, and use the +/- buttons until the display reads 24 minutes. Add 6 minutes for each additional pound of chicken over 4 pounds; for example, make it 30 minutes for 5 pounds.

recipe continues

5. When the cooker beeps to let you know it's finished, let it naturally come down from pressure until the display reads LO:10. Switch the pressure knob from the SEALING to the VENTING position. Use caution while the steam escapes—it's hot.

6. Open the cooker and check the internal temperature of your chicken with a meat thermometer. It should read about 165°F.

7. To crisp the skin and give the bird that golden look, place it under the broiler on high for 10 minutes or until golden brown.

creamy tuscan chicken with sun-dried tomatoes

• **I love how the sun-dried tomatoes in this recipe blend into the lusciously creamy sauce (which reduces dairy by using coconut milk). Serve over a spinach salad or over gluten- or grain-free pasta for a delicious and balanced meal.**

2 (8-ounce) boneless, skinless chicken breasts, thinly sliced

Sea salt

Black pepper

2 tablespoons extra-virgin olive oil

1 medium red onion, thinly sliced

1 cup chopped baby spinach

1/4 cup canned full-fat coconut milk or coconut cream

1 teaspoon garlic powder

1 teaspoon dried basil

1/2 teaspoon dried oregano

1/4 teaspoon dried thyme

1/2 cup grated parmesan cheese

1/2 cup sun-dried tomatoes

1. Lightly season the chicken with salt and pepper.

2. Preheat the pressure cooker using the SAUTE function and press the button until the display panel reads MORE. When the display panel reads HOT, add the oil, chicken, and onion. Sauté until the chicken begins to lose its color and the onion begins to become translucent, about 5 minutes.

3. Add the spinach, coconut milk, garlic powder, basil, oregano, thyme, cheese, and tomatoes; **do not stir.**

4. Put the lid on the cooker. Press the CANCEL button. Using the display panel, select the MANUAL/PRESSURE COOK function, high pressure, and use the +/- buttons until the display reads 2 minutes.

5. When the cooker beeps to let you know it's finished, let it naturally come down from pressure until the display reads LO: 20. Switch the pressure knob from the SEALING to the VENTING position. Use caution while the steam escapes—it's hot.

6. Open the cooker. Stir to combine all the ingredients. Press the CANCEL button and then program the cooker to SAUTE again. Let the sauce thicken, 2 to 3 minutes. Then press CANCEL. Serve warm.

savory barbecued chicken sliders

1 medium red onion, thinly sliced

2 (8-ounce) boneless, skinless
   chicken breasts

Sea salt

Black pepper

1 cup Homemade Barbecue Sauce
   (recipe follows)

8 Grain-Free Garlic Biscuits
   (page 185)

serves 4 to 6 • Sliders on Hawaiian rolls used to be a staple during game days at our house. But those rolls are so heavily processed and packed with sugar, it's definitely not worth it. I came up with this alternative that we're all just crazy for. Serve this yummy barbecued chicken sandwiched between my garlic herb biscuits and you'll have them shouting "Touchdown!" Or, for a lower-carb option, serve the chicken atop a leafy green salad dressed with Homemade Ranch Dressing (page 98).

1. Layer the onion slices on the bottom of a pressure cooker; this will help prevent the chicken from sticking.

2. Lightly season the chicken with salt and pepper. Lay the chicken on top of the onion slices.

3. Drizzle ½ cup of the barbecue sauce over the chicken.

4. Place the lid on the cooker and make sure the pressure knob is in the SEALING position. Using the display panel, select the MANUAL function, high pressure, and use the +/- buttons until the display reads 25 minutes.

5. When the cooker beeps to let you know it's finished, let it naturally come down from pressure until the display reads LO:13. Switch the pressure knob from the SEALING to the VENTING position. Use caution while the steam escapes—it's hot.

6. Open the lid of the cooker. Remove and shred the chicken. Add the remaining ½ cup barbecue sauce and stir to coat all the pieces. Serve the chicken sandwiched between halved biscuits.

recipe continues

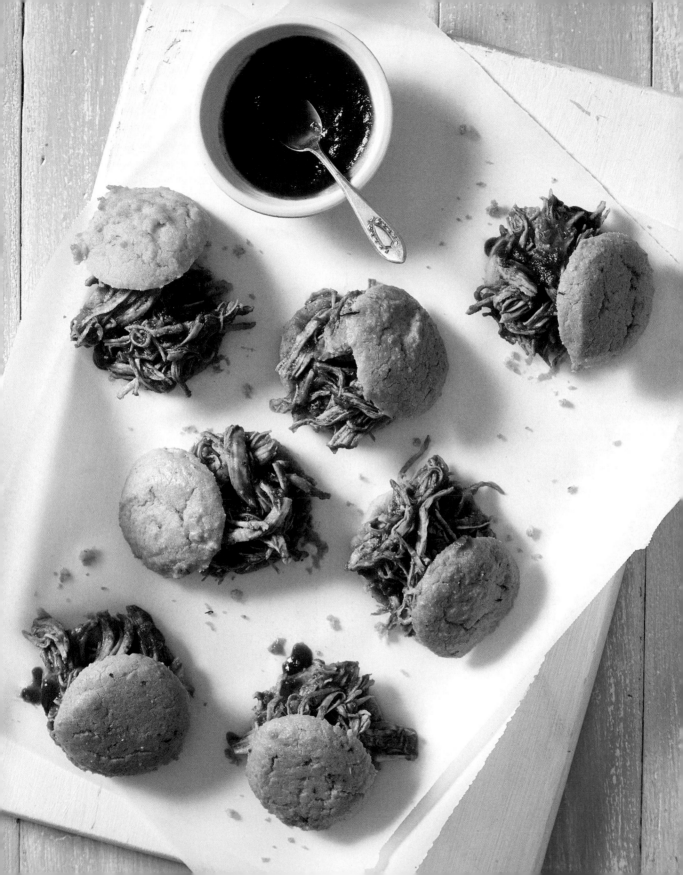

homemade barbecue sauce

makes 2 cups • When I started getting really savvy with my label reading, I realized that most store-bought versions of barbecue sauce were full of a highly processed form of sugar known as high-fructose corn syrup or simple corn syrup. These are both known to cause fatty liver disease and both should be banished from your home. This homemade sauce is a great alternative that you can feel secure in serving to your children. (It will keep in the refrigerator for up to 2 weeks or can be frozen for up to 6 months.)

1 (15-ounce) can organic tomato sauce

1/4 cup organic raw honey

1/3 cup red wine vinegar

2 tablespoons organic tomato paste

1 tablespoon low-sodium Worcestershire sauce

2 teaspoons liquid smoke

1 teaspoon sea salt

1 teaspoon dried minced onion

1/2 teaspoon chili powder

Combine all the ingredients in a saucepan over medium heat. Bring to a boil and then reduce the heat and simmer for 20 minutes, or until the sauce has thickened to desired consistency.

shredded beef tacos

2 pounds boneless beef stew meat or beef tips

3 teaspoons ground cumin

2 teaspoons chili powder

2 teaspoons dried minced onion

1 teaspoon sea salt

1 teaspoon black pepper

1/2 teaspoon cayenne

2 tablespoons extra-virgin olive oil

1 medium onion, thinly sliced

1 red bell pepper, cored, seeded, and thinly sliced

4 garlic cloves, thinly sliced

6 organic 6-inch corn tortillas

1 tablespoon avocado oil

serves 6 • **The pressure cooker has magical powers when it comes to cooking beef. It packs in the flavor and makes the meat fall apart. This shredded beef comes out so so juicy and flavorful that you don't even need salsa (and this is coming from a salsa fiend!). These tacos are a surefire hit for any Taco Tuesday.**

1. Season the beef with the cumin, chili powder, onion, salt, black pepper, and cayenne.

2. Preheat a pressure cooker using the SAUTE function. When the display panel reads HOT, add the oil and seasoned beef. Brown the meat on all sides, about 5 minutes.

3. Add the onion, bell pepper, and garlic. Sauté for 1 to 2 minutes more.

4. Place the lid on the cooker and make sure the pressure knob is in the SEALING position. Using the display panel, select the MEAT/STEW function, high pressure, and use the +/- buttons until the display reads 35 minutes.

5. Warm the tortillas in a skillet with the avocado oil. Keep them warm.

6. When the cooker beeps to let you know it's finished, switch the pressure knob from the SEALING to the VENTING position, administering a quick release. Use caution while the steam escapes—it's hot.

7. Open the cooker and serve the filling alongside the warm tortillas, so everyone can form individual tacos.

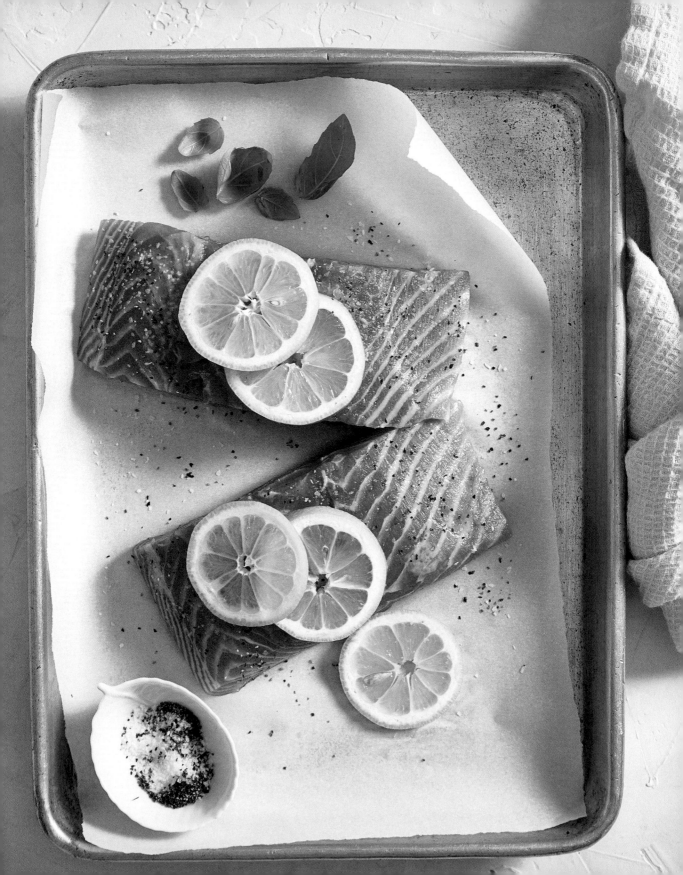

lemon basil *salmon*

1/4 to 1/2 cup fresh basil

2 (8-ounce) fillets wild-caught salmon

1/2 teaspoon sea salt

1/4 teaspoon black pepper

1/2 lemon, thinly sliced

serves 4 • Okay, I admit it. I'm not a huge fish lover, but I know it's good for me—all those healthy omega-3s! Surprisingly, though, I absolutely love this salmon! The fish flavor is very mild and the lemon basil offsets it well. So even if you wrinkle your nose at most fish dishes, give this one a try. You may just be surprised. Serve with Steamed Frozen Veggies (page 170) or a salad for a tasty, healthy meal.

1. Place 1/2 cup water and the basil in a pressure cooker. Set the trivet inside. Place the salmon skin side down on the trivet. Lightly sprinkle the fillets with the salt and pepper, then top with lemon slices.

2. Place the lid on the cooker and make sure the pressure knob is in the SEALING position. Using the display panel, select the STEAM function, high pressure, and use the +/- buttons until the display reads 3 minutes.

3. When the cooker beeps to let you know it's finished, switch the pressure knob from the SEALING to the VENTING position, administering a quick release. Use caution while the steam escapes—it's hot.

4. Open the cooker and remove the fish. Serve the fillets, dividing them into portions.

classic pot roast

serves 6 to 8 • **Traditionally, for a pot roast to come out tender and flavorful, it had to slowly cook in the oven for hours. With the pressure cooker, the cooking time is reduced to one hour, even if the roast is frozen—and it still comes out as tender and flavorful as expected.**

1 (4-pound) boneless beef
    rump roast

1 tablespoon black pepper

1 tablespoon extra-virgin olive oil

1 cup beef, chicken, or vegetable
    broth, homemade (pages 220–21)
    or store-bought

1 large onion, thinly sliced

4 garlic cloves, crushed

2 cups diced celery (about 4 stalks)

2 cups baby carrots

2 cups cubed sweet potatoes
    (1 to 2 medium)

2 teaspoons sea salt

2 teaspoons garlic salt

1 tablespoon organic tomato paste

1. Preheat a pressure cooker using the SAUTE function. Rub the meat with the pepper. When the display panel reads HOT, add the oil and brown the roast on all sides, about 5 minutes per side.

2. Add the broth and stir to dissolve the meat bits on the bottom of the cooker. Toss in the onion and garlic.

3. Place the lid on the cooker and make sure the pressure knob is in the SEALING position. Using the display panel, press the CANCEL button, then select the MANUAL/PRESSURE COOK function, high pressure, and use the +/- buttons until the display reads 60 minutes.

4. When the cooker beeps to let you know it's finished, switch the pressure knob from the SEALING to the VENTING position, administering a quick release. Use caution while the steam escapes—it's hot.

5. Working quickly, open the lid and add the celery, carrots, and sweet potatoes.

6. Place the lid back on the cooker and make sure the pressure knob is in the SEALING position. Using the display panel, press the CANCEL button, then select the MANUAL/PRESSURE COOK function, high pressure, and use the +/- buttons until the display reads 5 minutes.

7. When the cooker beeps to let you know it's finished, switch the pressure knob from the SEALING to the VENTING position, administering a quick release. Use caution while the steam escapes—it's hot.

8. Open the cooker and remove the vegetables and roast. Place them on a platter and salt to taste. Let the roast rest for about 15 minutes before cutting.

9. Using the display panel, press the CANCEL button, then select the SAUTE function. The liquid in the pot will begin to boil.

10. Add the tomato paste, the remaining teaspoon sea salt, and remaining teaspoon garlic salt. Let the sauce cook for about 10 minutes, to reduce slightly.

11. Slice the roast and pour the sauce over the roast and veggies, then serve.

classic meatloaf

serve 4 to 6 • **It may be classic, but there's nothing boring about this meatloaf. It's super-moist and full of flavor (and if you're not a fan of sweet in your savory, don't worry; you won't notice the apple at all). Serve it with a green salad or roasted veggies for a well-rounded meal your family will love.**

for the meatloaf:

1 pound lean grass-fed ground beef or turkey

1 cup gluten-free bread crumbs

½ cup finely chopped apple

½ cup finely chopped onion

½ cup Homemade Ketchup (page 225) or store-bought (without high-fructose corn syrup)

1 egg

1 tablespoon organic Dijon mustard

3 teaspoons dried parsley

1 teaspoon dried thyme

½ teaspoon garlic powder

½ teaspoon sea salt

¼ teaspoon black pepper

for the glaze:

¼ cup Homemade Ketchup (page 225) or store-bought (without high-fructose corn syrup)

½ tablespoon coconut aminos

⅛ teaspoon black pepper

1½ teaspoons chili powder

Pinch of ground chipotle chiles

1. Coat with cooking spray a small baking dish or loaf pan that can fit inside your pressure cooker.

2. Place the meatloaf ingredients in a bowl and mix well. Gather and shape into a loaf and place in the prepared pan.

3. In a small bowl, mix the glaze ingredients. Pour over the meatloaf, then cover the pan with foil.

4. For the potatoes, place the broth in the bottom of the pressure cooker, then set the potatoes in the cooker and add the trivet. Set the pan with the meatloaf on top of the trivet.

5. Place the lid on the cooker and make sure the pressure knob is in the SEALING position. Using the display panel, select the MANUAL/ PRESSURE COOK function, high pressure, and use the +/- buttons until the display reads 35 minutes.

6. When the cooker beeps to let you know it's finished, switch the pressure knob from the SEALING to the VENTING position, administering a quick release. Use caution while the steam escapes—it's hot.

7. Remove the lid and lift out the meatloaf onto a platter and allow it to rest for 5 minutes.

for the mashed potatoes:

¹/₂ cup chicken broth, homemade (page 220) or store-bought

4 red potatoes, quartered

¹/₂ teaspoon sea salt

1 tablespoon ghee

8. Thicken the glaze left in the pan by placing the baking pan under the broiler for a couple of minutes.

9. Remove the potatoes from the cooker and place in a large bowl. Add the salt and ghee, and, using an immersion blender, blend until smooth and creamy.

10. Slice the meatloaf, drizzle with the additional glaze, and serve with the potatoes.

shepherd's *pie*

1 large head of cauliflower, cored and cut into large florets

1/2 teaspoon garlic powder

2 teaspoons minced garlic

2 1/2 teaspoons sea salt

1 tablespoon olive oil

1 medium onion, diced

1 medium carrot, shredded

1 medium zucchini, shredded

1 teaspoon chili powder

1 tablespoon low-sodium Worcestershire sauce

1 to 1 1/2 pounds ground turkey

3/4 cup Mozzarella cheese (optional)

serves 8 • **This shepherd's pie is a bit different from the traditional. For one thing, it uses cauliflower instead of potatoes as a topping, making it lower in carbs. And it incorporates lean protein and tons of veggies instead of lamb, all the while maintaining the comfort touch of the original. It's a great, complete meal for chilly nights.**

1. Add 1 cup water to a pressure cooker. Place the trivet inside. Put the cauliflower on the trivet.

2. Using the display panel, select the MANUAL/ PRESSURE COOK, high pressure, function. Use the +/- buttons to select 3 minutes.

3. When the cooker beeps to let you know it's finished, switch the pressure knob from the SEALING to the VENTING position, administering a quick release. Use caution while the steam escapes—it's hot.

4. Open the cooker and remove the cauliflower, drain, then place it in a bowl. Add the garlic powder and 1 teaspoon of the salt, and blend with an immersion blender until smooth; these will be your mashed "potatoes."

5. Preheat the oven to 350°F.

6. Heat the oil in a large skillet over medium heat. Add the onion and remaining 2 teaspoons minced garlic. Sauté until the onion begins to soften and becomes translucent, about 5 minutes. Add the carrot, zucchini, remaining

recipe continues

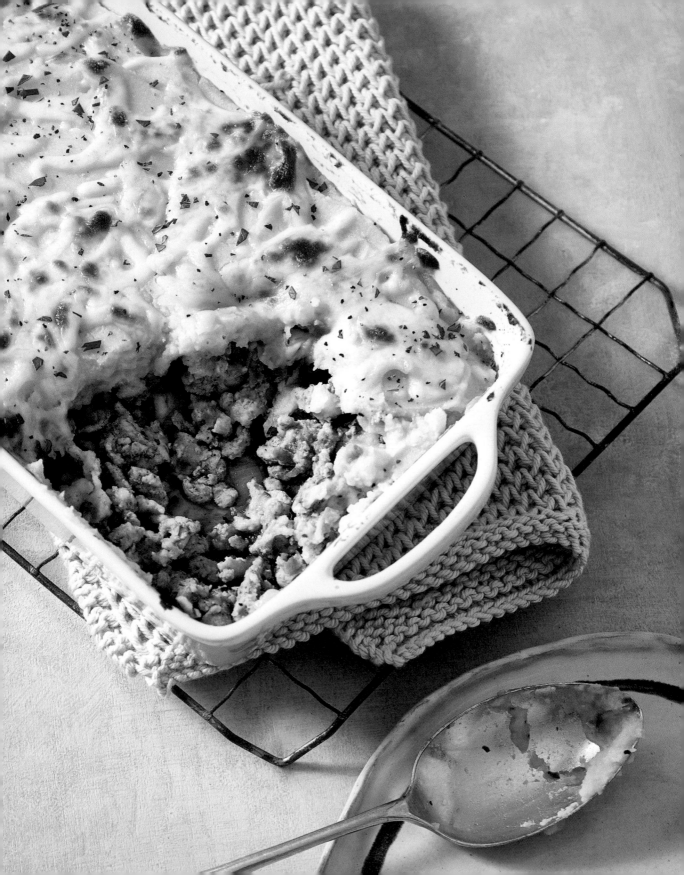

1½ teaspoons salt, the chili powder, and Worcestershire sauce. Sauté for a few minutes, then add the turkey.

7. Sauté the turkey, breaking it up and mixing with the vegetables, until all the liquid evaporates, about 10 minutes. If the liquid doesn't completely evaporate after the turkey has cooked, use a slotted spoon to transfer the turkey mixture without the liquid to a broiler-safe 8 × 8 × ½-inch glass baking dish.

8. Top with the mashed cauliflower and sprinkle with the Mozzarella, if using. Bake for 25 to 30 minutes, or until heated through.

9. Transfer the baking dish to the broiler for a couple of minutes so the cheese starts to bubble and brown on top.

classic tostadas

1 cup dried pinto beans

³/₄ cup water

¹/₄ cup chopped onion

¹/₂ cup chopped fresh cilantro

1 teaspoon sea salt

¹/₂ teaspoon cayenne

6 to 12 organic 6-inch corn tortillas

1 head of romaine lettuce, chopped

¹/₄ head of red cabbage, shredded

2 ripe medium tomatoes, diced

Salsa of choice

serves 4 to 6 • **These tostadas are my favorite meal ever. I love to serve them topped with my favorite hot sauce, El Pato. And here's the kicker: this entire meal can take as little as 10 minutes to prepare if you've premade the beans. Make the beans ahead of time or in a pinch use canned beans, chop all the veggies, and let everyone build his or her own tostada!**

1. Place the pinto beans in a bowl, cover with water, and let soak for 8 hours or overnight.

2. Rinse and drain the beans. Place the beans in a pressure cooker and cover with the ¾ cup water, the onion, cilantro, salt, and cayenne.

3. Place the lid on the cooker and make sure the pressure knob is in the SEALING position. Using the display panel, select the MANUAL/PRESSURE COOK function, high pressure, and use the +/- buttons until the display reads 12 minutes.

4. When the cooker beeps to let you know it's finished, let it naturally come down from pressure, 35 to 40 minutes. Switch the pressure knob from the SEALING to the VENTING position. Use caution while the steam escapes—it's hot.

5. Open the cooker and puree the beans with an immersion blender, or use a potato masher and mash them by hand.

6. Preheat the oven to 400°F. Spray a baking sheet with coconut oil spray and arrange the tortillas on it without overlapping. Bake for 2 minutes on each side or until golden.

7. Spread the beans on the tostada shells. Then layer the romaine, cabbage, and tomatoes, and drizzle with salsa.

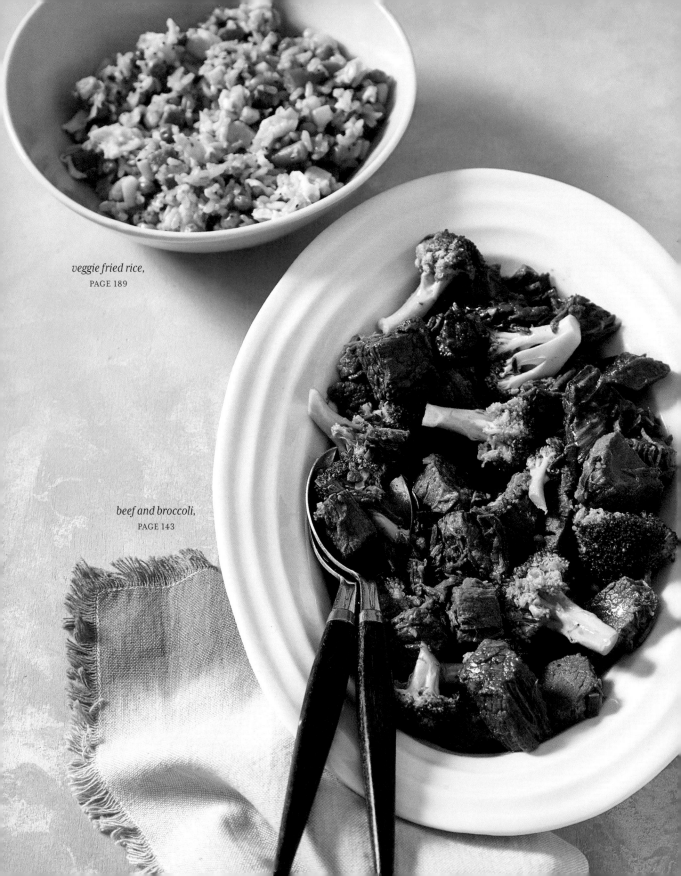

veggie fried rice,
PAGE 189

beef and broccoli,
PAGE 143

beef *and* broccoli

1 tablespoon extra-virgin olive oil

2 pounds boneless beef stew meat, cubed

1 medium onion, thinly sliced

1 tablespoon garlic powder

2 teaspoons sea salt

½ teaspoon black pepper

⅓ cup coconut aminos

1 teaspoon grated fresh ginger

1 tablespoon agave nectar

1 tablespoon arrowroot powder

2 pounds broccoli florets

serves 4 to 6 • **I'm a Chinese takeout kind of girl, but most Chinese restaurants use MSG and flavor enhancers in their recipes. Using a pressure cooker to make this classic dish at home is a cinch, and you won't have to worry about any harmful ingredients! Serve with Veggie Fried Rice (page 189) for a perfect combo.**

1. Preheat a pressure cooker using the SAUTE function. When the display panel reads HOT, add the oil, meat, onion, garlic powder, salt, and pepper. Sauté until the meat has browned on all sides, about 5 minutes.

2. Place the lid on the cooker and make sure the pressure knob is in the SEALING position. Using the display panel, press the CANCEL button, then select the MEAT/STEW function, high pressure, and use the +/- buttons until the display reads 35 minutes. If your cooker doesn't have the MEAT/STEW function, select the MANUAL/PRESSURE COOK function.

3. Combine the coconut aminos, ginger, and agave in a bowl.

4. When the cooker beeps to let you know it's finished, let it naturally come down from pressure until the display reads LO:15. Switch the pressure knob from the SEALING to the VENTING position. Use caution while the steam escapes—it's hot.

5. Remove the lid and press the CANCEL button. Select the SAUTE function, stir in the arrowroot, coconut aminos sauce, and the broccoli. Cook for a few minutes to thicken the sauce while the broccoli becomes tender.

6. Remove the beef and veggies and serve.

skinny enchiladas

for the sauce:

1 (15-ounce) can organic tomato sauce

1 tablespoon chili powder

1 teaspoon ground cumin

1/2 teaspoon garlic powder

1/4 teaspoon dried oregano

1/4 teaspoon sea salt

Pinch of ground cinnamon

4 organic 6-inch corn tortillas

1 pound ground beef, cooked and seasoned with 1/4 cup Taco Seasoning (page 231)

2 cups cooked black beans, homemade (page 226) or canned, rinsed and drained

1 large avocado, sliced

1 Roma (plum) tomato, diced

1 1/2 cups grated cheddar cheese (optional)

note: You can also bake this in your oven at 350°F for 30 minutes.

serves 6 • **These family-favorite enchiladas are screaming with flavor. They evolved in an interesting way. We've gone many summers without the use of an AC system because my husband and I gravitate toward older homes that predate central air. So I developed this pressure cooker recipe for when it's too boiling hot to turn on the oven.**

1. In a medium bowl, whisk together the sauce ingredients.

2. Using a 6-cup baking dish that can fit inside your pressure cooker, begin layering the ingredients. Spread a thin layer of enchilada sauce, then add a tortilla, some of the beef, some black beans, some avocado slices, and the cheese, if using. Repeat the layers three more times, reserving a few avocado slices for garnish. Cover with foil.

3. Put 1 cup water in a pressure cooker. Place the trivet in the cooker and add the dish of enchiladas.

4. Place the lid on the cooker and make sure the pressure knob is in the SEALING position. Using the display panel, select the MANUAL/PRESSURE COOK function, high pressure, and use the +/- buttons until the display reads 10 minutes.

5. When the cooker beeps to let you know it's finished, switch the pressure knob from the SEALING to the VENTING position, administering a quick release. Use caution while the steam escapes—it's hot.

6. Remove the foil. The cheese will be melted; if you want the top to crisp up, place the dish under the broiler for a few minutes. Serve topped with the diced tomato and remaining avocado slices.

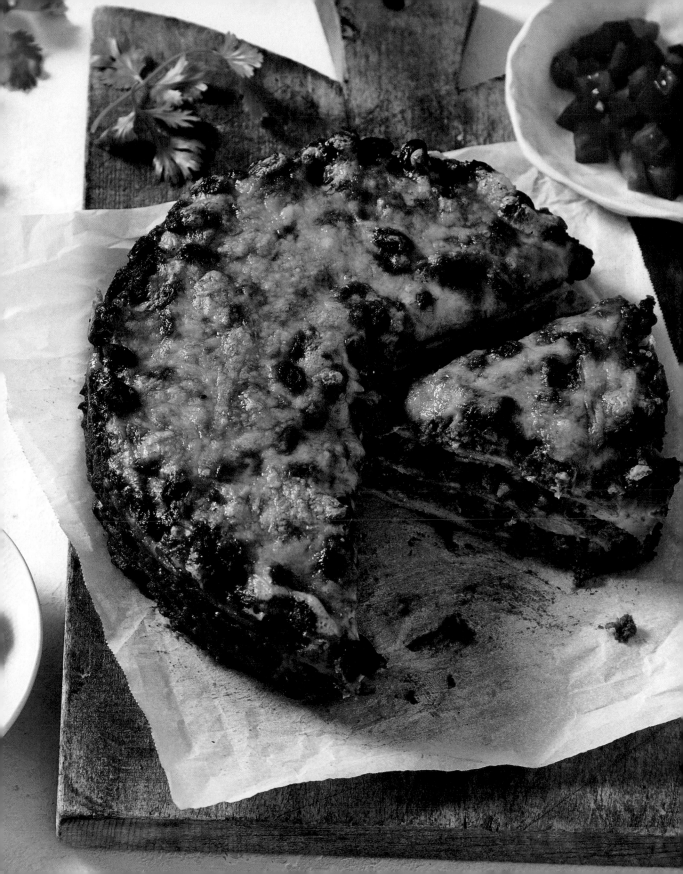

spicy stuffed peppers

serves 4 to 6 • **These peppers are stuffed with ground meat and cooked to perfection in the pressure cooker. This is a big meal in a little package, offering the holy trinity of clean eating: fat, fiber, and protein. This meal will leave everyone feeling satisfied.**

1 jalapeño, diced (seeds removed if you prefer less spicy)

1 medium onion, diced

1 pound ground meat of choice

¼ cup taco seasoning, homemade (page 231) or store-bought

Dash of cayenne

8 ounces salsa or picante sauce of choice

½ cup cooked rice or quinoa

4 bell peppers, any color, tops and seeds removed

1. Preheat the pressure cooker using the SAUTE function. When the display panel reads HOT, add the jalapeño and onion and dry-sauté until the onion becomes tender and translucent, about 5 minutes. Add the beef and brown it until it is about three-fourths done. Add the taco seasoning and cayenne.

2. Press the CANCEL button on the display panel. Drain off any grease and transfer the beef mixture to a bowl.

3. Place the liner back into the pressure cooker and add 1 cup water, then place the trivet inside.

4. Add the salsa and rice to the beef mixture and mix well. Use this to stuff the peppers, packing it into each tightly. Arrange the stuffed peppers on the trivet.

5. Place the lid on the cooker and make sure the pressure knob is in the SEALING position. Using the display panel, select the MANUAL/PRESSURE COOK function, high pressure, and use the +/- buttons until the display reads 12 minutes.

6. When the cooker beeps to let you know it's finished, let it naturally come down from pressure until the display reads LO:10. Switch the pressure knob from the SEALING to the VENTING position. Use caution while the steam escapes—it's hot.

7. Open the cooker and lift out the peppers; serve.

turkey
nuggets
and
fish sticks

¼ cup avocado oil

¼ cup coconut flour

1½ tablespoons arrowroot powder

½ teaspoon sea salt

¼ teaspoon dry mustard

¼ teaspoon black pepper

1 egg

½ tablespoon Homemade Almond Milk (page 223) or store-bought

1 pound ground turkey or 1 pound salmon fillet, skin removed and flesh cut into thin strips

serves 4 • **Serve this surf-and-turf combo with either Honey Mustard Dressing (page 109), Homemade Barbecue Sauce (page 130), or Homemade Ranch Dressing (page 98).**

1. Heat a skillet over medium heat, and add the oil.

2. Meanwhile, combine the coconut flour, arrowroot powder, salt, mustard, and pepper in a bowl.

3. In another bowl, whisk the egg and almond milk together.

4. Take a small piece of ground turkey and form a little "nugget-type" patty. Dip both sides of first the turkey nuggets and then the salmon strips in the egg mixture and dredge both in the flour mixture.

5. Add batches of the nuggets to the skillet and sauté over medium/medium-low heat, turning them when they brown and get crisp, 2 to 3 minutes on each side. Transfer the cooked nuggets to a paper towel–lined plate and keep warm while you similarly cook the salmon strips.

6. Serve the nuggets and fish strips while still hot.

PIZZAS, PASTAS, and BURGERS

kale and chicken-sausage alfredo *pizza*

1 tablespoon extra-virgin olive oil

2 chicken sausages, thinly sliced

1 cup chopped kale

1 tablespoon balsamic vinegar

¼ cup 5-Ingredient Dairy-Free Alfredo Sauce (page 157)

1 unbaked Grain-Free Pizza Crust (page 218), on parchment

serves 2 to 3 • **This dairy-free, grain-free pizza will blow your mind. It's so dynamite, it doesn't need cheese or a traditional pizza crust. Those things would only weigh you down! This scrumptious Italian treat will convert even the biggest clean-eating critic.**

1. Preheat the oven to 425°F.

2. Heat a skillet over medium heat and add the oil and sausage. Sauté until the sausage is lightly browned, about 5 minutes, then add the kale and vinegar. Continue to sauté until the kale wilts, another 5 to 10 minutes.

3. Spread the alfredo sauce on the pizza dough. Top with the sausage-kale mixture.

4. With the pizza still on the parchment, transfer to a baking sheet or pizza stone and bake for 11 minutes, or until the edges begin to turn golden.

note: Crust comes out better on a preheated pizza stone.

barbecued chicken *pizza*

serves 2 to 3 • **My sister worked at a pretty popular pizza place in North Texas. One of our favorite pizzas from that restaurant was a BBQ chicken pizza. So this recipe was inspired by all those yummy lunch visits with my sister, but here it is 100 percent grain and dairy free!**

1 (8-ounce) boneless, skinless chicken breast, cut into bite-size pieces

1/2 teaspoon sea salt

1/4 teaspoon black pepper

1 tablespoon extra-virgin olive oil

1/4 medium red onion, thinly sliced

1/4 cup Homemade Barbecue Sauce (page 130)

1 unbaked Grain-Free Pizza Crust (page 218), on parchment

1 1/2 tablespoons grated raw cashews

1. Preheat the oven to 425°F.

2. Season the chicken with the salt and pepper.

3. Heat a skillet over medium heat and add the oil, chicken, and onion. Sauté until the chicken is lightly browned and the onion begins to caramelize.

4. Spread the sauce on the pizza crust. Top with the chicken-onion mixture and sprinkle with the cashews.

5. Keeping the pizza on the parchment, slide it onto a baking sheet or pizza stone and bake for 11 minutes, or until the edges begin to turn golden.

note: Crust comes out better on a preheated pizza stone.

mediterranean vegetable pizza

½ cup chopped spinach

¼ medium red onion, thinly sliced

¼ cup diced yellow bell pepper

¼ cup white button mushrooms

½ tablespoon diced pitted Kalamata olives

¼ cup organic tomato sauce

1 unbaked Grain-Free Pizza Crust (page 218), on parchment

1 teaspoon garlic powder

½ teaspoon sea salt

1½ tablespoons grated raw cashews

serves 2 to 3 • Pizza is a great vehicle for getting more vegetables into your children. I like to set up a "pizza bar" on pizza night. Instead of one big pizza, I cut the dough into fifths and we do individual pan pizzas. Everyone gets to choose his or her own veggies. And for some reason, if the kids make their own pizzas, they eat ten times the veggies they would have otherwise. For individual pizzas, adjust the baking time to 9 minutes.

1. Preheat the oven to 425°F.

2. Heat a skillet over medium heat and add the spinach, onion, bell pepper, mushrooms, and olives. Sauté until the vegetables soften and the spinach wilts, about 5 minutes.

3. Spread the tomato sauce on the pizza dough. Sprinkle with the garlic powder and salt. Top with the vegetable mixture and sprinkle with the cashews.

4. Keeping the pizza on the parchment, slide it onto a baking sheet or pizza stone and bake for 11 minutes, or until the edges begin to turn golden.

note: Crust comes out better on a preheated pizza stone.

zoodles with basil pesto and sun-dried tomatoes

1/3 cup extra-virgin olive oil

1 cup fresh basil

1/4 cup pine nuts

1 garlic clove

2 medium zucchini

1/4 cup minced sun-dried tomatoes packed in olive oil

2 tablespoons grated cashews

1/4 teaspoon sea salt

Pinch of black pepper

serves 4 to 6 • **Sometimes it's nice to prepare something that doesn't require cooking at all. This delicious dish is so fresh and colorful that it cheers me up just to prepare it—and then I feel even better eating it. You will need a spiralizer to make it, though. This is one of my favorite recipes in the whole book. Simplicity is key to success.**

1. Place the oil, basil, pine nuts, and garlic in a high-powered blender and process until smooth.

2. Spiralize the zucchini. I like mine thin, so I use the 2 mm blade.

3. Toss the zucchini with the pesto and top with the sun-dried tomatoes and cashews. Season with the salt and pepper to taste.

· · · · · · · · ·

note: Filled with healthy fats, grated cashews taste like parmesan cheese—soft and melty and kind of salty. I started out making a spreadable cashew cheese, which is how I developed this idea of grating cashews as a substitute for grated parmesan.

*zoodles with basil pesto
and sun-dried tomatoes,*
PAGE 153

mediterranean vegetable pizza.
PAGE 152

spaghetti squash *with* *dairy-free* *alfredo* *sauce*

serves 6 • When I was growing up, a fancy dinner was a jar of Alfredo sauce tossed with some quick-cooking tortellini. Super-high in carbohydrates and full of dairy, these meals were a surefire way to pack on the pounds. I wanted to come up with a dairy-free Alfredo sauce that we could enjoy without feeling guilty afterward. This version is made with cashews; I know it sounds crazy, but it works! Toss with some shredded spaghetti squash and you have a high-protein, creamy, delectable substitute. Be sure to select a squash that fits inside your pressure cooker!

1 medium spaghetti squash that will fit inside your pressure cooker

5-Ingredient Dairy-Free Alfredo Sauce (recipe follows)

....

note: If your spaghetti squash is smaller than indicated above, decrease the cooking time by 10 minutes. If you like your spaghetti squash al dente, decrease the cooking time by 15 minutes.

1. Put 1 cup water in the bottom of a pressure cooker. Place the trivet inside and put your spaghetti squash on top.

2. Place the lid on the cooker and make sure the pressure knob is in the SEALING position. Using the display panel, select the MANUAL/PRESSURE COOK function, high pressure, and use the +/- buttons until the display reads 30 minutes.

3. When the cooker beeps to let you know it's finished, switch the pressure knob from the SEALING to the VENTING position, administering a quick release. Use caution while the steam escapes—it's hot.

4. Remove the squash and let cool on the counter for 15 minutes. Cut in half, spoon out the seeds in the middle, and discard the seeds. Using a fork and holding one half of the squash, pull shreds outward from the peel to make squash "spaghetti." Repeat with the remaining half.

5. Place the squash in a bowl and add the sauce. Stir to coat well and serve.

5-ingredient dairy-free alfredo sauce

makes 3 cups

1 cup raw cashews

2 cups water

2 tablespoons unfortified nutritional yeast

2 teaspoons sea salt

3 garlic cloves

Place all the ingredients in a high-powered blender. Blend until everything is smooth and creamy and the sauce thickens and becomes steaming hot, about 8 minutes.

one-pot spaghetti with meat sauce

1 medium onion, diced

3 garlic cloves, minced

1 cup white button mushrooms, diced (optional)

1¼ pounds lean ground beef

1 tablespoon dried minced onion

2 teaspoons dried oregano

2 teaspoons garlic powder

2 teaspoons dried basil

1 teaspoon sea salt

½ teaspoon dried thyme

¼ teaspoon black pepper

¼ teaspoon red pepper flakes

8 ounces gluten- or grain-free pasta of choice

2 (15-ounce) cans organic tomato sauce

1 (15-ounce) can organic diced tomatoes

serves 6 to 8 • **I've been told that my marinara is the best in the world. It's only half mine, though, as my mom used to make a similar spaghetti sauce. Now I make it for my own kids, but I'm able to cut the cooking time and the number of dirty dishes by doing it all in one pot and using my pressure cooker!**

1. Preheat the pressure cooker using the SAUTE function. When the display panel reads HOT, add the diced onion, garlic, and mushrooms, if using. Dry-sauté until the vegetables begin to become translucent and stick to the bottom of the pan, about 5 minutes.

2. Add the beef and lightly brown, about 5 minutes, then add the onion, oregano, garlic powder, basil, salt, thyme, black pepper, and red pepper flakes. Stir and continue to cook the meat until well browned, about 3 minutes more.

3. Spread the mixture to cover the bottom of the cooker. Break the pasta into thirds, if long, and layer on top of the meat. Pour in the tomato sauce and place the diced tomatoes on top. **Do not stir**; if the sauce comes into contact with the bottom of the cooker, it can scorch.

4. Place the lid on the cooker and make sure the pressure knob is in the SEALING position. Using the display panel, press the CANCEL button, then select the MANUAL/PRESSURE COOK function, high pressure, and use the +/- buttons until the display reads 10 minutes.

5. When the cooker beeps to let you know it's finished, switch the pressure knob from the SEALING to the VENTING position, administering a quick release. Use caution while the steam escapes—it's hot.

6. Open the lid and stir. Serve warm.

eggplant parmesan

serve 4 to 6 • **This dish can be grain free depending on the pasta you use. I love Ancient Harvest brand, and their quinoa pasta is great in this dish. And yes, I know it's unconventional to use pasta in eggplant parm! You can leave it out and serve with a small side salad.**

1 medium-large eggplant, cut into bite-size pieces

1 egg, whisked till frothy

1/2 cup gluten-free panko bread crumbs

1 teaspoon garlic powder

1 teaspoon chopped fresh parsley

1 tablespoon extra-virgin olive oil

1/2 cup chicken or vegetable broth, homemade (pages 220–21) or store-bought

8 ounces gluten-free pasta of choice

1 (15-ounce) can organic tomato sauce

1/2 tablespoon dried minced onion

1 1/2 teaspoons dried oregano

1/2 teaspoon dried basil

1/4 teaspoon dried thyme

1/4 teaspoon sea salt

1/4 teaspoon black pepper

1 cup freshly grated parmesan cheese, plus more for serving

1/2 cup fresh basil, for serving

1. Preheat the pressure cooker using the SAUTE function, then press the SAUTE button until the display panel reads MORE.

2. Toss the eggplant with the egg, then add the bread crumbs, garlic powder, and parsley. Toss to coat.

3. When the cooker display panel reads HOT, add the oil and eggplant. Brown the eggplant on one side, then flip over to brown on the other side, about 2 minutes on each side.

4. Add the broth and pasta on top of the eggplant layer. Then add the tomato sauce. **Do not stir;** if the sauce touches the bottom of the pressure cooker, there is a chance it could scorch. Add the onion, oregano, dried basil, thyme, salt, and pepper. Top with the cheese.

5. Place the lid on the cooker. Using the display panel, select the CANCEL button. Then press the MANUAL/PRESSURE COOK function, high pressure, and use the +/- buttons until the display reads 5 minutes.

6. When the cooker beeps to let you know it's finished, switch the pressure knob from the SEALING to the VENTING position, administering a quick release. Use caution while the steam escapes—it's hot.

7. Open the cooker and stir. Serve warm with a fresh sprinkling of cheese and fresh basil.

summer shrimp scampi with zoodles and chickpeas

1½ to 2 pounds jumbo shrimp, shells removed and deveined

2 tablespoons ghee

5 garlic cloves, minced

½ cup chicken broth, homemade (page 220) or store-bought

¾ teaspoon sea salt

⅛ teaspoon red pepper flakes

2 medium zucchini

½ cup cooked chickpeas, homemade (page 227) or canned, rinsed and drained

½ cup chopped fresh parsley or basil

½ cup grape tomatoes, cut in half

2 tablespoons fresh lemon juice (optional)

serves 4 to 6 • Zucchini noodles, a.k.a. zoodles, are a brilliant way to lighten up the traditionally carb-heavy shrimp scampi with pasta. And it comes together in a flash. This dish has all the flavor you love, plus an extra dose of healthy veggies.

1. Place the shrimp, ghee, garlic, broth, salt, and red pepper flakes in a pressure cooker.

2. Place the lid on the cooker and make sure the pressure knob is in the SEALING position. Using the display panel, select the STEAM function, high pressure, and use the +/- buttons until the display reads 1 minute.

3. When the cooker beeps to let you know it's finished, switch the pressure knob from the SEALING to the VENTING position, administering a quick release. Use caution while the steam escapes—it's hot.

4. Spiralize the zucchini (I like mine thin so I use the 2 mm blade).

5. Open the cooker and place the shrimp in a bowl. Toss the shrimp with the zucchini, chickpeas, parsley, tomatoes, and lemon juice, if using. Use the broth left in the bottom of the cooker as dressing. Adjust seasoning to taste.

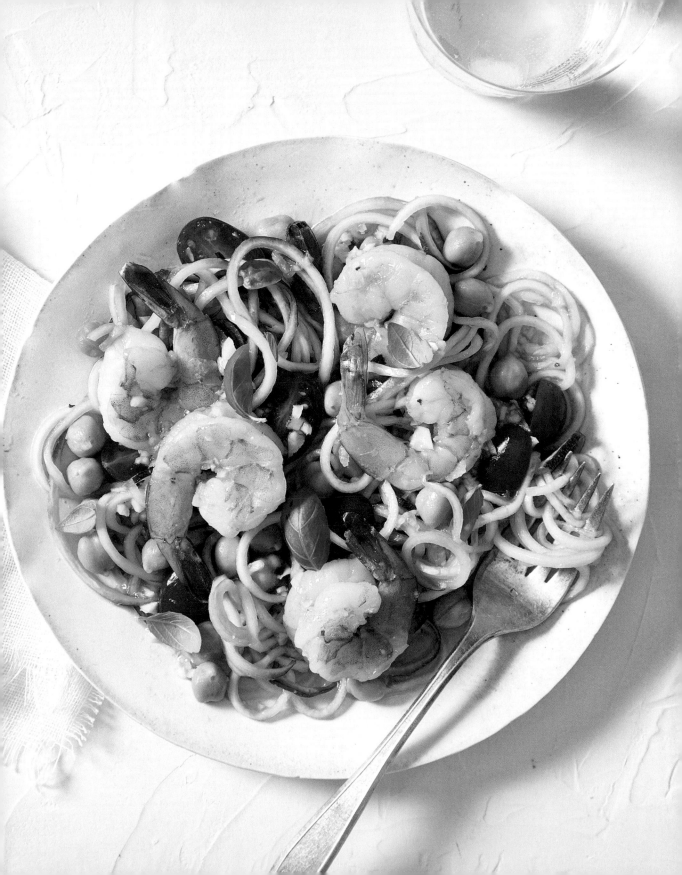

vegetable lasagna

1 cup raw cashews

1 teaspoon sea salt

3 tablespoons water

2 tablespoons extra-virgin olive oil

1 tablespoon fresh lemon juice

1 (15-ounce) can organic diced tomatoes

1 tablespoon dried minced onion

½ cup fresh parsley or basil

½ teaspoon red pepper flakes

½ teaspoon dried basil

2 to 3 medium zucchini

2 cups chopped kale or spinach

note: If you have a nut allergy, replace the vegan cheese with ricotta.

serves 4 to 6 • My lasagna recipe has evolved a lot over the years. It began as a jarred ragu mixture combined with ricotta, mozzarella, and pasta. Then I began substituting vegetables for the pasta and homemade sauce for the jarred. Eventually not even the cheese was left. We make it now with vegan cashew cheese, and you know what? We adjusted just fine! It's different from traditional lasagna, but it's so yummy and flavorful.

1. Place the cashews, ½ teaspoon of the salt, the water, oil, and lemon juice in a high-powered blender and blend on high until the mixture resembles cream cheese. Transfer to a bowl.

2. Add the tomatoes, onion, parsley, red pepper flakes, dried basil, and remaining ½ teaspoon salt to the blender or a food processor. Pulse until combined.

3. Cut zucchini lengthwise into very thin slices to fit your 6-cup baking dish.

4. In a 6-cup baking dish that fits inside your pressure cooker, layer the ingredients. Begin with about one-fourth of the tomato sauce, then add one-fourth of the zucchini, one-fourth of the cashew mixture, and one-fourth of the kale. Repeat, making three more layers. Cover with foil.

5. Put 1 cup water in a pressure cooker. Place the trivet inside and put the dish of lasagna on top.

6. Place the lid on the cooker and make sure the pressure knob is in the SEALING position. Using the display panel, select the MANUAL/PRESSURE COOK function, high pressure, and use the +/- buttons until the display reads 10 minutes.

7. When the cooker beeps to let you know it's finished, switch the pressure knob from the SEALING to the VENTING position, administering a quick release. Use caution while the steam escapes—it's hot.

8. Remove the dish from the cooker and let the lasagna cool for 10 to 15 minutes before serving.

skinny mac and no cheese

2 cups water

1/3 cup diced carrot

1/4 cup arrowroot powder

1/4 cup unfortified nutritional yeast

1 tablespoon ghee

1 1/2 teaspoons sea salt

8 ounces gluten- or grain-free elbow or shell pasta

serves 4 • **Mac and cheese is always in demand at my house, and if you have kids, it probably is at yours, too. This no-cheese version's surprise serving of carrots and clean ingredients, means you won't mind your kids eating it as often as they want it.**

1. Place the water, carrot, arrowroot powder, nutritional yeast, and ghee in a high-powered blender. Blend on medium-high until combined. The mixture will be very watery; that's okay.

2. Transfer the mixture to a pressure cooker. Follow by placing the pasta on top.

3. Place the lid on the cooker and make sure the pressure knob is in the SEALING position. Using the display panel, select the MANUAL function, high pressure, and use the +/- buttons until the display reads 5 minutes.

4. When the cooker beeps to let you know it's finished, switch the pressure knob from the SEALING to the VENTING position, administering a quick release. Use caution while the steam escapes—it's hot.

5. Open the cooker and serve.

sun-dried tomato and basil chickpea *patties*

2 cups cooked chickpeas, homemade (page 227) or canned, rinsed and drained

1 egg

¼ cup fresh basil

1 tablespoon minced sun-dried tomatoes in olive oil

1 teaspoon sea salt

½ teaspoon dried oregano

Pinch of red pepper flakes

2 tablespoons extra-virgin olive oil

6 large leaves of butterhead lettuce

1 Roma (plum) tomato, sliced

Garlic Vinaigrette (recipe follows)

serves 4 • **This is a surprising Mediterranean spin on the veggie burger, which I like to serve wrapped in butterhead lettuce and topped with a slice of juicy tomato.**

1. Place the chickpeas, egg, basil, sun-dried tomatoes, salt, oregano, and red pepper flakes in a food processor and pulse 8 to 10 times. Transfer to a bowl and form 6 small patties.

2. Heat a skillet over medium heat and add the oil. Place the patties in the skillet without crowding; you may need to use 2 skillets or do it in 2 batches.

3. Cook the patties until lightly browned, about 5 minutes, then flip and cook for 3 more minutes on the other side.

4. Wrap each patty in a lettuce leaf and top with a tomato slice. Drizzle on some dressing and serve.

garlic vinaigrette

makes ¼ cup

3 large garlic cloves, minced

1½ teaspoons balsamic vinegar

¼ cup extra-virgin olive oil

Place all the ingredients in a jar and shake well.

10-minute turkey burgers

1 pound ground turkey

1 egg

½ cup gluten-free old-fashioned rolled oats

½ cup chopped baby spinach

½ cup chopped green onions or chives

1 tablespoon dried minced onion

1 teaspoon sea salt

Black pepper

3 tablespoons extra-virgin olive oil

Burger fixins' of choice

serves 4 to 6 • **Yup, just 10 minutes! These lean burgers pack a stealthy dose of spinach, and you can serve them over a salad for a super-healthy meal or on grain-free buns for a more classic burger experience. If burgers mean ketchup to you, make the Homemade Ketchup (page 225). However you have your burger, your taste buds will thank you.**

1. Place the turkey, egg, oats, spinach, green onions, onion, salt, and pepper to taste in a bowl. Mix gently to combine. Form into 6 larger or 8 smaller patties.

2. Heat a skillet that has a lid over medium-high heat and add the oil. Place the patties in the skillet a few at a time; you may need to do this in 2 batches. Sauté the patties until lightly browned, about 5 minutes, then flip and cover with the lid, cooking an additional 3 minutes.

3. Serve topped with your favorite fixins'.

10-minute turkey burgers,
PAGE 166

sweet potato french fries,
PAGE 182

VEGGIES
and
OTHER SIDES

steamed frozen *veggies*

16 ounces frozen vegetable blend, with cauliflower, broccoli, carrots, etc.

Sea salt

Black pepper

Grated parmesan cheese or grated cashews (optional)

serves 4 to 6 • **When I had a lot of weight to lose, this was my #1 go-to lunch. I would steam an entire basketful of veggies and eat that for lunch with a protein on the side (egg, natural turkey, chicken); it was a nutrient-packed lunch that kept me full. My philosophy was to keep it simple, and that worked.**

1. Put 1 cup water into a pressure cooker. Place a steamer basket inside. Add the frozen mixed vegetables to the basket.

2. Place the lid on the cooker and make sure the pressure knob is in the SEALING position. Using the display panel, select the STEAM function, low pressure, and use the +/- buttons until the display reads 0.

3. When the cooker beeps to let you know it's finished, switch the pressure knob from the SEALING to the VENTING position, administering a quick release. Use caution while the steam escapes—it's hot.

4. Open the cooker. Sprinkle the veggies with a little salt and pepper and serve. If desired, add a liberal sprinkling of grated parmesan or grated cashews. YUM!

. . . .

tip: Make sure you release the pressure and take off the lid right away so you don't overcook the veggies.

maple-glazed *carrots*

4 cups chopped carrots, into bite-size pieces

¾ cup chicken broth, homemade (page 220) or store-bought

¼ cup pure maple syrup

1 teaspoon low-sodium Worcestershire sauce

serves 4 to 6• **This is a traditional, simple side dish. Instead of brown sugar, we use pure maple syrup for the sweetness, and the Worcestershire sauce gives it a savory flavor as well. This is a perfect slimmed-down twist on an old favorite.**

1. Place all the ingredients in a pressure cooker.

2. Place the lid on the cooker and make sure that the pressure valve is in the SEALING position. Using the display panel, select the STEAM function, high pressure, and use the +/- buttons until the display reads 1 minute.

3. When the cooker beeps to let you know it's finished, press the CANCEL button and remove the lid.

4. Select the SAUTE function and let the carrots boil with the lid off for 5 minutes or until half of the liquid has evaporated. Remove and serve.

tip: If your cooker does not have a steam function, use the MANUAL or PRESSURE COOK function.

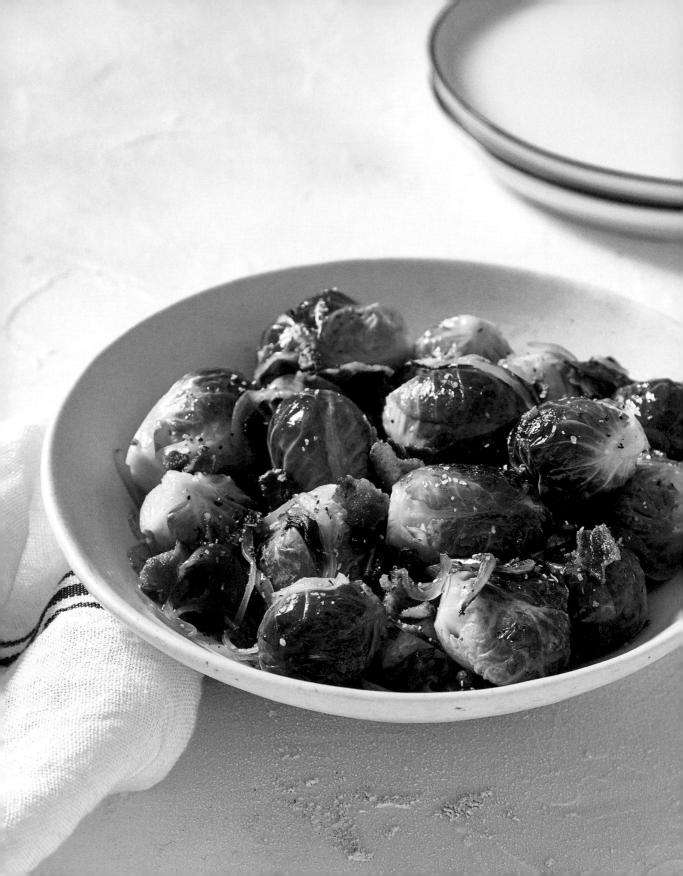

savory bacon brussels sprouts

1 (12-ounce) package nitrate-free bacon, chopped into bite-size pieces

1/2 medium onion, thinly sliced

1 tablespoon ghee

1 pound Brussels sprouts, trimmed

Sea salt

Black pepper

serves 4 to 6 • **We don't eat a lot of pork in our house, but we can't get enough bacon! And while you could technically use turkey bacon, do yourself a favor and use real bacon if you can. It took me a long time to like Brussels sprouts, but I can eat this by the bowl!**

1. Preheat the pressure cooker using the SAUTE function, then press the SAUTE button until the display panel says MORE. When the display panel says HOT, add the bacon and sauté until crisp, about 15 minutes. Remove from the cooker and drain on a paper towel.

2. Add the onion and ghee to the bacon grease in the cooker. Continue to sauté until the onion begins to become translucent, about 3 minutes.

3. Add the Brussels sprouts and toss with the onion.

4. Place the lid on the cooker and make sure the pressure knob is in the SEALING position. Using the display panel, press the CANCEL button and select the MANUAL/PRESSURE COOK function. It does not matter if the knob is in the pressure or sealing position; the pot will not come to pressure. Using the display panel, select the STEAM function, high pressure, and use the +/- buttons until the display reads 2 minutes.

5. When the cooker beeps to let you know it's finished, open the lid and toss the Brussels sprouts with the bacon. Add salt and pepper to taste and serve.

lemon garlic- butter *artichokes*

2 globe artichokes

2 tablespoons extra-virgin olive oil

1 tablespoon ghee

8 garlic cloves, minced

1 teaspoon minced fresh or dried parsley

1 teaspoon fresh lemon juice

serves 2 to 4 • **I had no idea how to eat an artichoke the first time I bought one. I watched a YouTube video on what to do. I'm so glad I did. Now it's one of my kids' favorite vegetables.**

1. Cut the stems off of the artichokes with a knife and trim the tips using kitchen shears.

2. Place 1 cup water in a pressure cooker. Place the trivet or a steamer rack inside and set the artichokes on top.

3. Put the lid on the cooker and make sure the pressure knob is in the SEALING position. Using the display panel, select the MANUAL/PRESSURE COOK function, high pressure, and use the +/- buttons until the display reads 10 minutes.

4. While the artichokes are steaming, combine the oil and ghee in a small saucepan over low heat. When it begins to bubble and ripple, add the garlic, parsley, and lemon juice. Sauté for 1 to 2 minutes, no longer; garlic burns quickly.

5. When the cooker beeps to let you know it's finished, let it naturally come down from pressure for 13 minutes. The pin should drop around this time.

6. Remove the lid from the cooker, then remove the artichokes. Cut each in half if serving 4.

7. To eat an artichoke, pull off one leaf at a time, starting from the bottom, and dip it in the lemon-garlic butter. Place the leaf in your mouth and gently scrape the meat off the bottom using your teeth. Discard the rest. When you have eaten all the leaves, take a knife and cut around the thistle in the center; discard. Then cut the bottom into quarters and dip in the dressing to enjoy the heart (or bottom).

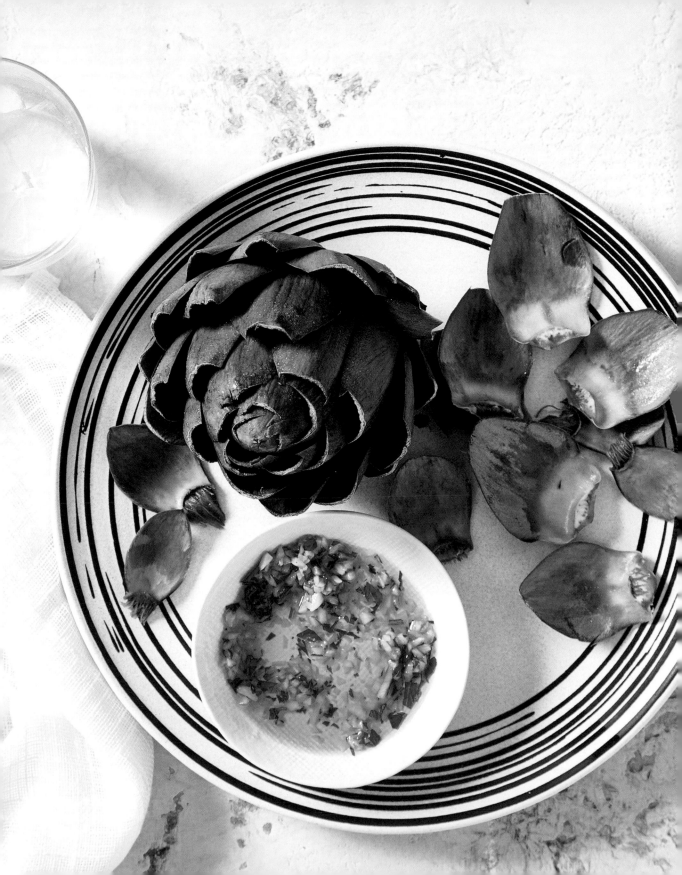

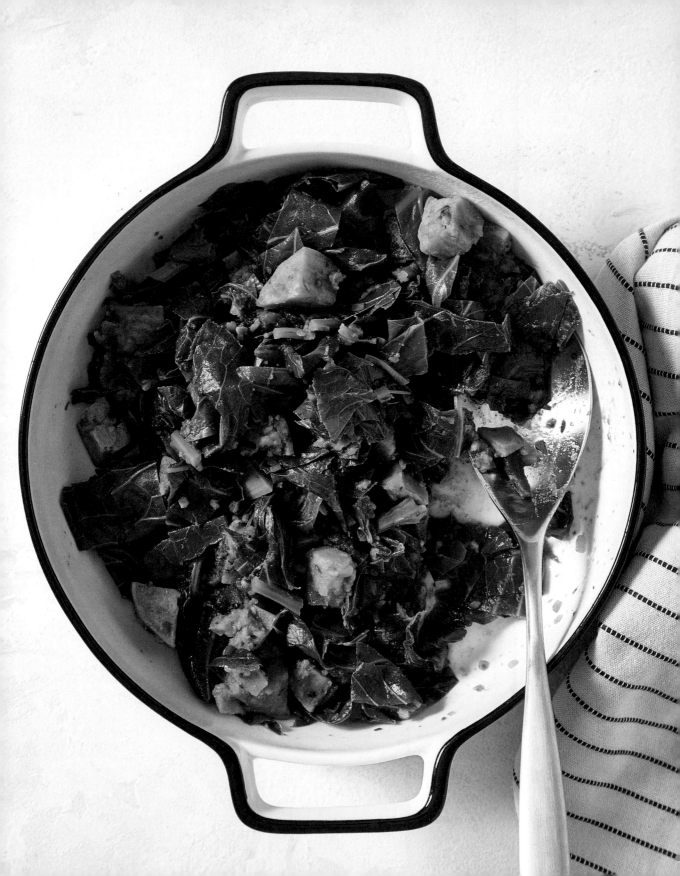

curried collard greens *with sweet potatoes*

2 bunches of collard greens, stems cut out and leaves cut into bite-size pieces

1 large sweet potato, cubed (about 2 cups)

1 (15-ounce) can organic fire-roasted diced tomatoes

1 tablespoon dried minced onion

1 teaspoon ground cumin

1 teaspoon dried oregano

1 teaspoon dried thyme

1/2 teaspoon curry powder

1/2 teaspoon ground turmeric

1/2 teaspoon sea salt

serves 4 to 6 • **The spices make this dish, and I love that I can get my kids to eat turmeric! Cooked collard greens contain 9 grams of protein per cup, so this is a complete meal. It's a great side dish as well, and can also be served for lunch.**

1. Layer the collard greens, sweet potato, and fire-roasted tomatoes in a pressure cooker. **Do not stir.** Sprinkle the onion, cumin, oregano, thyme, curry powder, turmeric, and salt over the top.

2. Place the lid on the cooker and make sure the pressure knob is in the SEALING position. Using the display panel, select the MANUAL/PRESSURE COOK function, high pressure, and use the +/- buttons until the display reads 10 minutes.

3. When the cooker beeps to let you know it's finished, let it naturally come down from pressure until the display reads LO:10. Switch the pressure knob from the SEALING to the VENTING position. Use caution while the steam escapes –it's hot.

4. Open the cooker and serve warm.

10-minute caramelized onions

1 large onion, thinly sliced

1 to 2 teaspoons extra-virgin olive oil

1/4 to 1/2 teaspoon balsamic vinegar

Sea salt

Black pepper

makes 1 cup • **Brady eats onions on everything! He loves these caramelized onions on top of his steak, chicken, or burger patties. If you're going to put these on steak or chicken breast, you can also add mushrooms when you cook the onions.**

1. Preheat a pressure cooker using the SAUTE function. Press the SAUTE button until the screen says MORE. When the display panel reads HOT, add all the ingredients and move them around with a wooden spoon, cooking until they are reduced, about 10 minutes.

2. Remove the onions and place in a bowl to serve at once or pack into a jar and refrigerate for future use.

easy beets

As many beets as desired, scrubbed and trimmed of greens and roots

yield varies • **A nutritional powerhouse, beets also make everything beautiful! Instead of using red or pink food dye, as some food producers do, you can use beets for a bright beautiful color without altering the taste of whatever you're making. Cook these ahead and store them in the fridge, ready for you to toss into smoothies or give a boost of nutrients and color to sauces.**

1. Pour 1 cup water into a pressure cooker. Place the trivet inside and set the beets on top.

2. Using the display panel, select the MANUAL/PRESSURE COOK function, high pressure, and use the +/- buttons until the display reads 25 minutes.

3. When the cooker beeps to let you know it's finished, let it naturally come down from pressure, about 10 minutes.

4. Open the lid carefully and remove the beets. Place them in a bowl and run each beet under running water as you slip the skins off. Pack them into jars or storage containers and store in the refrigerator until you're ready to use.

salty baked potatoes

3 pounds baby red potatoes

1/2 cup sea salt

6 cups water

serves 4 to 6 • **Cooking these potatoes in salted water makes them incredibly flavorful. If you have a salt craving, these are for you! You can add leftover chili, some ranch dressing or, better yet, combine some ranch dressing with some barbecue sauce for mega-flavor with your potatoes. Of course, they are just as great by themselves.**

1. Place all the ingredients in a pressure cooker.

2. Using the display panel, select the MANUAL/PRESSURE COOK function, high pressure, and use the +/- buttons until the display reads 2 minutes.

3. When the cooker beeps to let you know it's finished, let it naturally come down from pressure, about 12 minutes.

4. Open the lid carefully and remove the potatoes. Top with your favorite fixings and serve with a side salad.

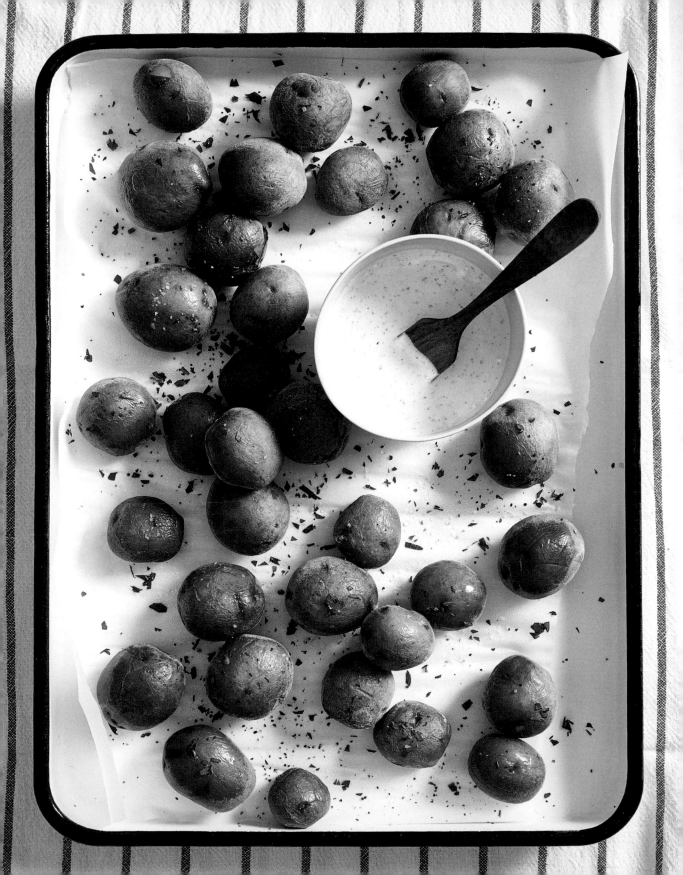

sweet potato *french fries*

1 pound sweet potatoes,
   cut into strips

2 tablespoons extra-virgin olive oil

1 teaspoon sea salt

serves 4 to 6 • **Super simple. Super easy. These are one of our favorite snacks. They can always curb even my worst fast-food cravings.**

1. Preheat the oven to 475°F.

2. Toss the sweet potatoes in a bowl with the oil and salt, then arrange on a baking sheet in a single layer.

3. Bake the potatoes for 20 to 25 minutes, or until browned and crisp. Serve at once.

southern-style *green beans*

6 slices turkey bacon (or nitrate-free regular bacon, if desired)

2 pounds green beans, trimmed and cut in half

2 cups vegetable or chicken broth, homemade (page 220) or store-bought

1 teaspoon sea salt

1 teaspoon dried minced onion

5 garlic cloves, minced

1/2 teaspoon black pepper

1/4 teaspoon red pepper flakes

Butter or ghee (optional)

serves 6 to 8 • **This is a down-home Southern side dish. When I lived in Texas, you couldn't go to someone's house without there being green beans in one form or another. Heavy cream is a foundation for many of the green bean recipes in the South, so instead of heavy cream, the vegetable or chicken broth makes this a low-calorie alternative.**

1. Preheat the pressure cooker using the SAUTE function, and press the SAUTE button until the display panel says MORE. When the display panel says HOT, add the bacon and sauté until crisp, about 15 minutes. Remove and set on a paper towel to drain.

2. Add the beans, broth, salt, onion, garlic, black pepper, and red pepper flakes to the cooker.

3. Place the lid on the cooker. Make sure the vent valve is in the SEALING position. Using the display panel, select the MANUAL/PRESSURE COOK function, low pressure, and use the +/- buttons until the display reads 5 minutes.

4. When the cooker beeps to let you know it's finished, switch the pressure knob from the SEALING to the VENTING position, administering a quick release. Use caution while the steam escapes—it's hot.

5. Remove the lid and add the bacon. Toss the beans, adding the butter (if using), then remove and serve.

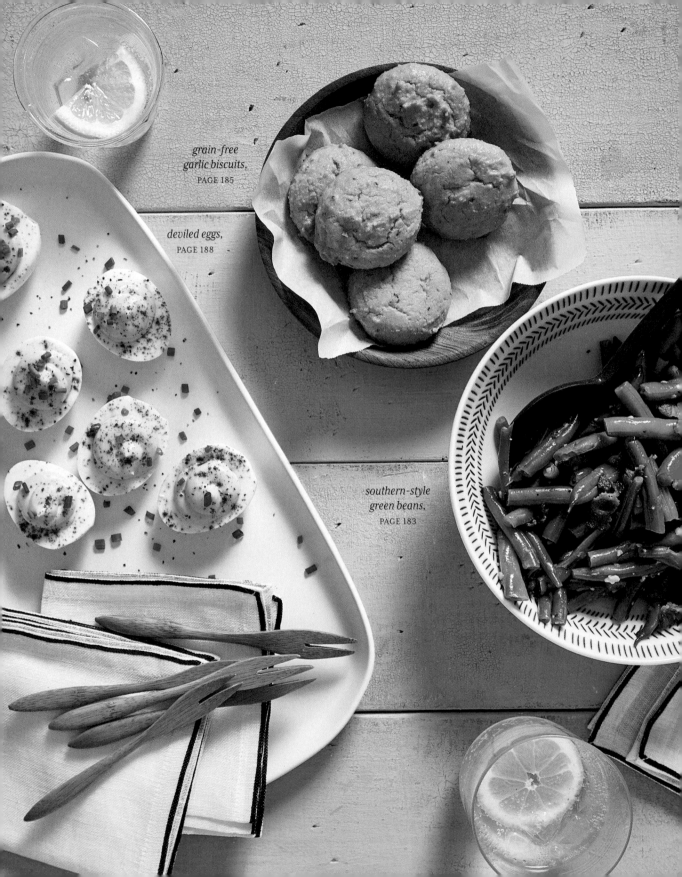

grain-free garlic biscuits,
PAGE 185

deviled eggs,
PAGE 188

southern-style green beans,
PAGE 183

grain-free garlic biscuits

2 tablespoons avocado oil

¾ cup (packed) almond flour

½ teaspoon garlic powder

¼ teaspoon dried parsley

¼ teaspoon sea salt

2 eggs

makes 8 biscuits • **These yummy biscuits are grain free and delicious served coupled with my Spicy Tomato Basil Soup (page 82) or cut in half and filled with Savory Barbecued Chicken (page 128).**

1. Preheat the oven to 350°F. Coat a baking sheet with cooking spray.

2. Place all the ingredients in a bowl and blend gently with a hand mixer.

3. Using a cookie scoop, transfer balls of the batter to the prepared baking sheet. You should have enough to form 8 balls.

4. Bake for 15 to 20 minutes, or until lightly browned and cooked through.

5. Transfer to a rack to cool slightly and serve warm.

dairy-free creamed corn

1 cup raw cashews

3 cups vegetable or chicken broth, homemade (pages 221 and 220) or store-bought

¼ cup unfortified nutritional yeast

1 teaspoon sea salt

¼ teaspoon black pepper

2 tablespoons fresh lemon juice

1 tablespoon apple cider vinegar

4 cups frozen corn kernels

6 slices turkey bacon (or nitrate-free regular bacon, if desired), cooked and crumbled

serves 10 • **Creamed corn is my signature Thanksgiving side dish, and so I'm responsible for bringing it to our big family dinner every year. This version uses cashew cheese instead of dairy, and it pleases everyone gathered around the holiday table.**

1. Place the cashews, 2 cups of the broth, the nutritional yeast, salt, pepper, lemon juice, and vinegar in a high-powered blender. Blend on high until smooth.

2. Place the corn in a pressure cooker. Cover with the cashew mixture and add the remaining 1 cup broth. **Do not stir**.

3. Put the lid on the cooker. Make sure the pressure knob is in the SEALING position. Using the display panel, select the MANUAL/PRESSURE COOK function, high pressure, and use the +/- buttons until the display reads 10 minutes.

4. When the cooker beeps to let you know it's finished, switch the pressure knob from the SEALING to the VENTING position, administering a quick release. Use caution while the steam escapes—it's hot.

5. Remove the lid and add the bacon right before serving. The creamed corn will thicken as it cools a bit. Remove from the cooker and serve.

hard-boiled *eggs*

6 to 12 eggs

yield varies • **This popular method of pressure-cooking eggs is known as the 5-5-5 method. I've been doing this for the last four years, and it's never steered me wrong. I highly recommend using the steamer/strainer basket instead of the trivet; it simplifies things a little.**

1. Add 1 cup water to a pressure cooker. Place a steamer basket or trivet inside and arrange the eggs carefully on top, making sure none are leaning against the side of the cooker.

2. Place the lid on the cooker and make sure the pressure knob is in the SEALING position. Using the display panel, select the STEAM function, high pressure, and use the +/- buttons until the display reads 5 minutes.

3. While the eggs cook, fill a bowl with ice cubes and water.

4. When the cooker beeps to let you know it's finished, let it come down naturally from pressure until the display reads LO:5. Switch the pressure knob from the SEALING to the VENTING position. Use caution while the steam escapes—it's hot.

5. Remove the lid and immediately remove the eggs, placing them one at a time into an ice bath to stop the cooking process. Let sit for 5 minutes before peeling.

deviled *eggs*

6 Hard-Boiled Eggs (page 187), peeled and rinsed

3 tablespoons Homemade Mayonnaise (page 224) or store-bought

2 teaspoons organic yellow mustard

Paprika, for sprinkling

makes 12 deviled eggs • **My dad is the master of deviled eggs—this is well known in our family and his eggs are requested at every family event. But he keeps his recipe a secret! After studying his method intently one Thanksgiving, I was able to replicate his delicious dish. This is a common snack or lunch in our home now. If we're eating these as a meal, I usually serve them with a side salad, veggie platter, and applesauce with them as well.**

1. Gently cut the eggs in half lengthwise. Remove the yolks and place in a bowl. Set the egg whites on a plate or a deviled egg dish.

2. Add the mayo and mustard to the egg yolks, using a fork to combine.

3. Spoon the mixture into the halved egg whites and sprinkle the tops with paprika.

veggie
fried rice

1 (16-ounce) package frozen mixed vegetables (carrots, peas, green beans, corn, etc.)

1½ cups brown rice

1 (13.5-ounce) can full-fat coconut milk

1 cup vegetable or chicken broth, homemade (pages 221 and 220) or store-bought

3 tablespoons dried minced onion

½ teaspoon sea salt

¼ teaspoon black pepper

6 to 8 eggs

½ tablespoon extra-virgin olive oil

Coconut aminos, for serving

serves 6 • **Brown rice is a great side dish to accompany a veggie-focused dinner, but every once in a while I enjoy it as a stand-alone meal. You have your fat, fiber, and protein all packed into this yummy classic takeout dish.**

1. Set the bag of frozen vegetables on the counter to start thawing.

2. Place the brown rice, coconut milk, broth, onion, salt, and pepper in a pressure cooker.

3. Place the lid on the cooker and make sure the pressure knob is in the SEALING position. Using the display panel, select the MULTIGRAIN function, high pressure, and use the +/- buttons until the display reads 28 minutes.

4. Meanwhile, crack the eggs into a bowl and whisk until fluffy.

5. Heat a skillet over medium heat and add the oil. Pour in the eggs and scramble until cooked through, about 5 minutes. Add the vegetables and stir to help them thaw.

6. When the cooker beeps to let you know it's finished, switch the pressure knob from the SEALING to the VENTING position, administering a quick release. Use caution while the steam escapes—it's hot.

7. Open the lid and add the egg-and-vegetable mixture. Stir to combine the rice with the eggs and veggies. Remove from the cooker and serve with coconut aminos.

spanish rice

1 cup brown rice

1½ cups water or broth

½ cup organic tomato sauce

½ cup El Pato or other mild red hot sauce or enchilada sauce of choice

1 cup ground meat of choice, cooked and seasoned with Taco Seasoning (page 231)

serves 4 to 6 as a side • **My aunt Kim is one of my greatest cooking inspirations because she always made it look so easy to prepare healthy meals for a family of seven. This is one of her staples, with my own little twist. It's a great potluck dish and simple to make a larger serving by doubling the recipe.**

1. Place the brown rice and water in a pressure cooker.

2. Place the lid on the cooker and make sure the pressure knob is in the SEALING position. Using the display panel, select the MANUAL/PRESSURE COOK function, high pressure, and use the +/- buttons until the display reads 28 minutes.

3. When the cooker beeps to let you know it's finished, switch the pressure knob from the SEALING to the VENTING position, administering a quick release. Use caution while the steam escapes—it's hot.

4. Open the cooker and stir in the tomato sauce, hot sauce, and meat. Remove from the cooker and serve.

cilantro lime *rice*

1 cup brown rice

2 cups vegetable broth, homemade (page 221) or store-bought

1/2 tablespoon avocado oil

2 garlic cloves, minced

1 lime, zested and juiced

1/3 cup chopped fresh cilantro

1/2 teaspoon sea salt

serves 4 as a side • **Chipotle anyone? The Chipotle restaurants are one of our favorite spots to stop when we're running around and need a bite to eat that's pretty healthy. This Cilantro Lime Rice was inspired by the rice in their delicious burrito bowls.**

1. Place the brown rice, broth, oil, garlic, and lime zest in a pressure.

2. Place the lid on the cooker and make sure the pressure knob is in the SEALING position. Using the display panel, select the MANUAL/PRESSURE COOK function, high pressure, and use the +/- buttons until the display reads 28 minutes.

3. When the cooker beeps to let you know it's finished, switch the pressure knob from the SEALING to the VENTING position, administering a quick release. Use caution while the steam escapes—it's hot.

4. Open the cooker and add the cilantro, salt, and lime juice. (Add the lime juice little by little until it suites your taste.) Remove from the cooker and serve.

DESSERTS,
DRINKS,
and
SHAKES

apple "pie" à la mode

• **This is a lighter version of homemade apple pie with dairy-free vanilla ice cream. It's warm and comforting, and will make your home smell like autumn!**

2 large red apples, cored, peeled, and sliced

1 tablespoon ghee or coconut oil

1 tablespoon pure maple syrup

1¹/₂ teaspoons ground cinnamon

¹/₄ teaspoon ground nutmeg

³/₄ cup gluten-free granola, plus more for serving

Pinch of sea salt

Dairy-free vanilla ice cream (page 209, variation of Peaches and Cream Ice Cream)

1. Place the apples in a pressure cooker and add in the ghee. Pour the maple syrup over top, then sprinkle with cinnamon and nutmeg. Add the granola and salt.

2. Place the lid on the cooker and make sure the pressure knob is in the SEALING position. Using the display panel, select the MANUAL/PRESSURE COOK function, high pressure, and use the +/- buttons until the display reads 5 minutes.

3. When the cooker beeps to let you know it's finished, switch the pressure knob from the SEALING to the VENTING position, administering a quick release. Use caution while the steam escapes—it's hot.

4. Open the lid and scoop out the apples. Serve with ice cream and a sprinkle of granola.

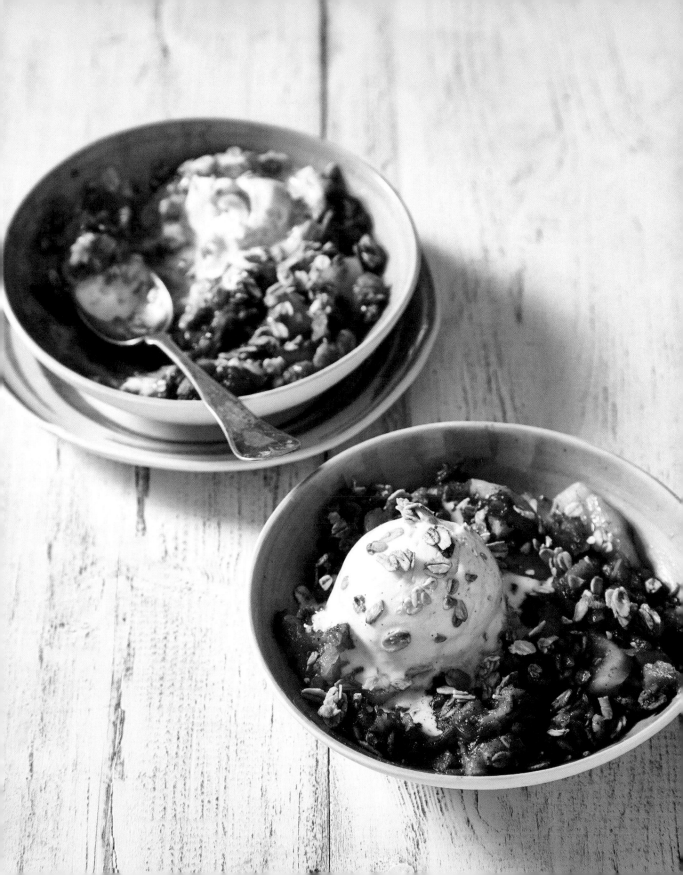

chocolate-covered mixed nut clusters

1 cup dairy-free chocolate chips

1 tablespoon ghee or coconut oil

2½ cups mixed nuts

Add-ins: dried cranberries or blueberries, sunflower seeds, pumpkin seeds

makes 20 ounces • **Chocolate with mixed nuts was one of my favorite go-to snacks while I was losing weight. I love to convert my pressure cooker into a double boiler to make my own little snack clusters. It satisfies the sweet tooth and it's easier than making them on the stovetop!**

1. Pour about 2 cups water in a pressure cooker and place inside a shallow 3-quart glass or stainless steel bowl, like a double boiler. The bottom of the bowl should not touch the water. Line a baking sheet with parchment.

2. Using the display panel, select the SAUTE function. Press the SAUTE button until the display says MORE.

3. Add the chocolate chips and ghee to the bowl. Whisk until the chocolate has melted, about 5 minutes. Using a rubber spatula, stir in the nuts and any add-ins.

4. Transfer silver-dollar-size clusters of chocolate to the prepared baking sheet.

5. Refrigerate for 1 hour. When hard, store in a glass container in the refrigerator for up to 6 months.

guilt-free brownies

1¼ cups cooked black beans, homemade (page 226) or canned, rinsed and drained

3 eggs

½ tablespoon pure vanilla extract

¼ teaspoon sea salt

3 tablespoons extra-virgin coconut oil

¼ cup raw unfiltered honey or pure maple syrup

3 tablespoons cacao powder

½ teaspoon baking powder

¼ teaspoon baking soda

¼ cup dairy-free chocolate chips

makes 10 • **Shhh, there are black beans in this recipe, but if you don't tell, no one will ever know! Black beans are a fantastic flour substitute. You can also substitute applesauce for the oil in this recipe to achieve even fewer calories and less fat. These are chocolatey, fudgy, and delicious.**

1. Place all the ingredients in a high-powered blender or a food processor and process until smooth.

2. Coat with cooking spray a 6-cup baking dish that fits inside your pressure cooker. Add the batter, spread out in the dish, and cover with foil.

3. Put the trivet in the pressure cooker, then pour in 1 cup water. Place the baking dish on the trivet.

4. Place the lid on the cooker and make sure the pressure knob is in the SEALING position. Using the display panel, select the MANUAL/PRESSURE COOK function, high pressure, and use the +/- buttons until the display reads 45 minutes.

5. When the cooker beeps to let you know it's finished, switch the pressure knob from the SEALING to the VENTING position, administering a quick release. Use caution while the steam escapes—it's hot.

6. Open the lid and wait 5 minutes for the brownies to cool, then cut into 10 pieces and transfer to a plate to enjoy!

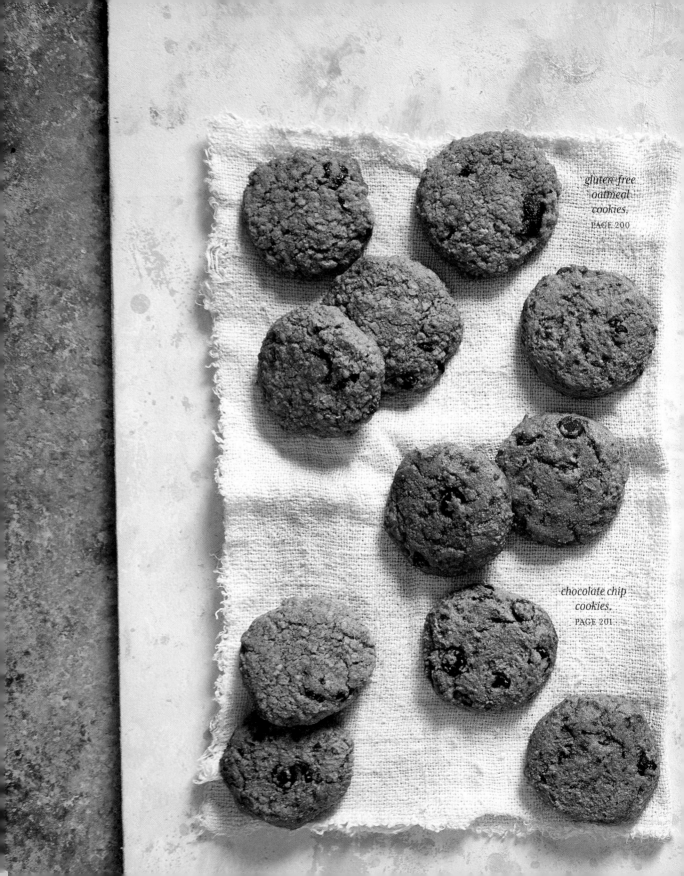

gluten-free oatmeal cookies, PAGE 200

chocolate chip cookies, PAGE 201

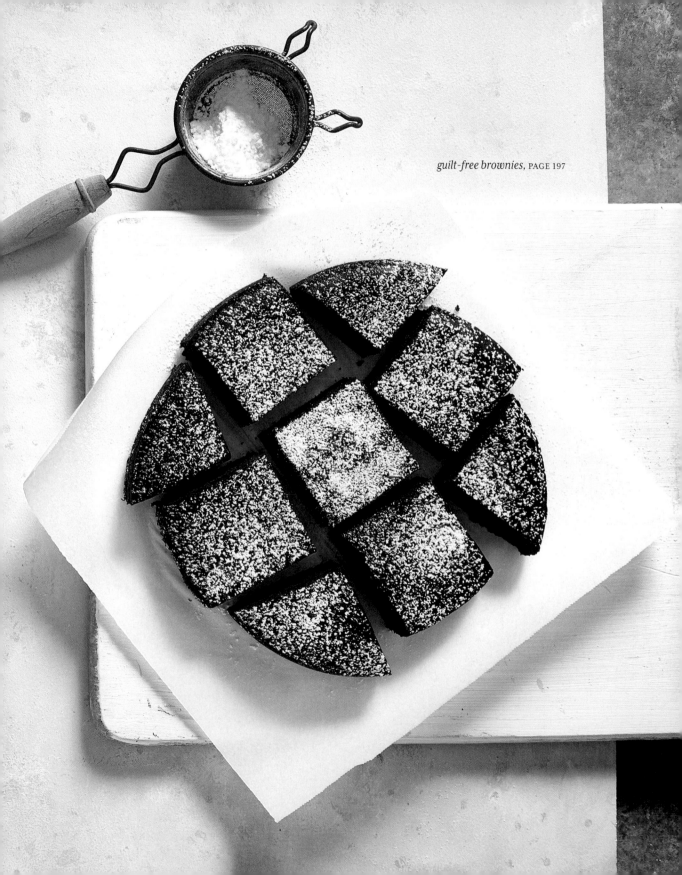

guilt-free brownies, PAGE 197

gluten-free oatmeal cookies

makes 16 cookies • My grandma has a traditional oatmeal cookie recipe that our entire family loves. But I adapted her recipe to fit our new gluten-free lifestyle. This is one of my boys' favorites, so I love that I can still make my grandma's, even if slightly modified. Take your pick of filling, whether raisins, chocolate chips, dried cranberries, or dried blueberries—they all work great!

1 cup gluten-free quick-cooking oats

1 cup (packed) almond flour

¼ cup organic raw honey

1 egg

2 tablespoons coconut oil, solid or melted

½ teaspoon baking soda

½ teaspoon ground cinnamon

Pinch of sea salt

1 teaspoon pure vanilla extract

¼ cup raisins, dairy-free chocolate chips, dried cranberries, or dried blueberries

1. Preheat the oven to 375°F. Lightly coat a cookie sheet with coconut oil spray.

2. Place all the ingredients, except for the raisins and other add-ins, in a bowl. Use a hand or a stand mixer to combine until smooth. Stir in the raisins, chocolate chips, or berries.

3. Using a 1½ tablespoon cookie scoop, form the dough into balls and place on the prepared sheet. Lightly press the tops until they flatten into ½-inch disks.

4. Bake for 8 to 10 minutes, or until golden and cooked through. Let cool a few minutes, then transfer to a rack to cool completely.

chocolate chip *cookies*

1 cup (packed) almond flour

2 tablespoons coconut sugar

1 tablespoon pure maple syrup

1 egg

1 teaspoon pure vanilla extract

¼ teaspoon baking soda

¼ teaspoon sea salt

¼ cup dairy-free chocolate chips

makes 10 cookies • **This is a lifestyle change, not a diet! Here, you just substitute the traditional ingredients with healthier alternatives and remember to control your portions. My tip? Freeze these cookies (and other desserts) in individual serving sizes so you're not tempted to eat them all at once.**

1. Preheat the oven to 350°F. Lightly coat a cookie sheet with coconut oil spray.

2. Place the flour, sugar, maple syrup, egg, vanilla, baking soda, and salt in a food processor. Process on high for 10 to 15 seconds, or until well combined. Stir in the chocolate chips.

3. Using a 1½ tablespoon cookie scoop, transfer the batter to the prepared sheet; you should get 10 balls. Press gently on the tops to flatten the balls into disks.

4. Bake for 10 minutes, or until lightly browned. Let cool slightly, then transfer the cookies to a rack to cool completely.

peanut butter *blondies*

2 cups cooked chickpeas, homemade (page 227), or canned, rinsed and drained

¼ cup organic peanut, almond, or sunflower butter

¼ cup organic raw honey

1 teaspoon pure vanilla extract

¼ teaspoon sea salt

¼ teaspoon baking powder

⅛ teaspoon baking soda

¼ cup dairy-free chocolate chips

makes 16 blondies • **These blondies are made with chickpeas! Using legumes instead of flour is one of my favorite ways to give our old favorites a healthy makeover, upping the protein and fiber content in the process. If you have a nut allergy, you can use a seed butter, like sunflower seed butter, to make this recipe as well.**

1. Preheat the oven to 350°F. Coat an 8-inch square baking dish with coconut oil.

2. Place all the ingredients, except the chocolate chips, in a food processor and blend until smooth. Your batter will be very thick and sticky, like brownie batter. Stir in the chocolate chips by hand.

3. Spread the batter into the prepared dish and smooth the top.

4. Bake for 35 minutes, or until lightly golden. Let cool briefly then cut into 16 pieces. Let cool before serving.

note: If using canned chickpeas, make sure that they don't have any salt added.

double chocolate *blender cake*

1 medium to large ripe banana

2 eggs

2 tablespoons coconut oil, melted or solid

2 tablespoons organic raw honey

3 tablespoons cacao powder

1 cup gluten-free old-fashioned rolled oats

1/2 cup (packed) almond flour

1 teaspoon baking soda

1 teaspoon pure vanilla extract

1/4 teaspoon sea salt

1/4 cup dairy-free chocolate chips

variation

If you prefer, this cake can be baked in the oven instead. Preheat the oven to 350°F and bake for 25 minutes, or until a toothpick inserted in the center comes out clean. Let cool for 5 minutes before flipping the cake over onto a cake stand for serving.

serves 8 to 10 • **This fluffy little cake tastes just like a chocolate cupcake. Light, airy, and gluten free, it has banana and honey instead of sugar for sweetness. I've given the instructions for cooking in a pressure cooker, but see also the oven alternative below.**

1. Coat a 6-cup Bundt pan with coconut oil spray.

2. Place all the ingredients in a high-powered blender and blend on high until the mixture forms a smooth batter. Pour the batter into the pan and cover with foil.

3. Pour 1 cup water into a pressure cooker. Place the pan on the trivet and gently lower it into the cooker.

4. Place the lid on the cooker and make sure the pressure knob is in the SEALING position. Using the display panel, select the MANUAL/PRESSURE COOK function, high pressure, and use the +/- buttons until the display reads 30 minutes.

5. When the cooker beeps to let you know it's finished, switch the pressure knob from the SEALING to the VENTING position, administering a quick release. Use caution while the steam escapes—it's hot.

6. Open the cooker and gently remove the cake. Allow it to cool for 5 minutes before flipping the cake over onto a cake stand and serving.

no-cheese cake *with* raspberry coulis

serves 10 • Cheesecake without the cheese? Yes, it can be done! I love a cheesecake that is creamy and tart, and not too heavy. This one is indulgent, but its ingredients are cleaner than what you'll find at a restaurant. And it is perfectly complemented by the Raspberry Coulis, made from fresh, whole berries.

for the crust:

¼ cup coconut flour

2 tablespoons (packed) almond flour

½ teaspoon ground cinnamon

¼ teaspoon baking soda

⅛ teaspoon sea salt

2 tablespoons coconut palm shortening

2 tablespoons organic raw honey

½ teaspoon pure vanilla extract

for the filling:

2 cups raw cashews

10 tablespoons unsweetened vanilla almond milk

1 teaspoon pure vanilla extract

¼ cup coconut sugar or raw organic sugar

2 tablespoons organic raw honey

1 teaspoon fresh lemon juice

Raspberry Coulis (recipe follows)

1. Coat with cooking spray a 7-inch baking dish that fits into your pressure cooker.

2. Combine the coconut flour, almond flour, cinnamon, baking soda, and salt in a food processor. Pulse to combine. Add the coconut shortening and pulse until the mixture resembles coarse, even crumbs. Add the honey and vanilla, and pulse just until the mixture is blended. Pour into the prepared dish. Using the back of a spoon, spread the mixture evenly across the dish and press gently to evenly cover the bottom of the dish and make a crust.

3. Combine all the filling ingredients in a high-powered blender. Process until smooth. Add the filling to the crust. Cover the top of the dish with foil.

4. Pour 1 cup water into a pressure cooker. Place the dish on the trivet and gently lower it into the cooker.

5. Place the lid on the cooker and make sure the pressure knob is in the SEALING position. Using the display panel, select the MANUAL/PRESSURE COOK function, high pressure, and use the +/- buttons until the display reads 35 minutes.

6. When the cooker beeps to let you know it's finished, switch the pressure knob from the SEALING to the VENTING position, administering a quick release. Use caution while the steam escapes—it's hot.

7. Open the lid and gently remove the cheesecake from the pressure cooker. Allow to cool for 5 minutes before serving with the raspberry coulis. Store leftovers in the refrigerator.

raspberry coulis

makes 1⅓ cups

8 ounces fresh raspberries

¼ cup pure maple syrup

1 tablespoon water

½ teaspoon fresh lemon juice

Puree the ingredients in a high-powered blender and serve on top of cheesecake.

gluten-free carrot cake

serves 8 to 10 • **Dense and rich, this cake is addictive. Make sure to put it away after you cut your slice or you will be tempted to eat until it's gone. The Dairy-Free Buttercream is literally the icing on the cake. Make sure to use a high-powered blender like a Vitamix for this recipe, as a regular blender will not work.**

1 egg

2 tablespoons ghee or coconut palm shortening

2 tablespoons pure maple syrup

3 tablespoons coconut sugar

1/3 cup unsweetened applesauce

1/4 teaspoon sea salt

3/4 teaspoon baking soda

1/2 teaspoon baking powder

1/2 teaspoon ground cinnamon

1/3 cup unsweetened vanilla almond milk or water

1/2 cup (packed) almond flour

1/2 cup gluten-free old-fashioned rolled oats

1/2 cup grated carrots (about 2 small)

1/4 cup pecans or walnuts, chopped

Dairy-Free Buttercream Frosting (recipe follows)

1. Coat with cooking spray a 6-cup square baking dish that fits inside your pressure cooker.

2. Place all the ingredients, except the carrots, pecans, and frosting, in a high-powered blender. Blend on high until smooth. Stir in the carrots and pecans, then pour into the prepared dish and cover the dish with foil.

3. Pour 1 cup water into the pressure cooker. Place the dish on the trivet and gently lower it into the cooker.

4. Place the lid on the cooker and make sure the pressure knob is in the SEALING position. Using the display panel, select the MANUAL/PRESSURE COOK function, high pressure, and use the +/- buttons until the display reads 35 minutes.

variation

If you prefer, this cake can be baked in the oven. Double the recipe and grease a 9-inch round cake pan. Preheat the oven to 350°F and bake for 35 minutes, or until a toothpick inserted in the center comes out clean. Let cool for 10 minutes, then invert and remove from the pan.

5. When the cooker beeps to let you know it's finished, switch the pressure knob from the SEALING to the VENTING position, administering a quick release. Use caution while the steam escapes—it's hot.

6. Open the lid and gently remove the carrot cake from the pressure cooker. Allow to cool for 10 minutes, then invert and remove from the dish. Let cool completely before frosting.

dairy-free buttercream frosting

makes ⅔ cup, enough for 1 small cake

1 cup soaked raw cashews, drained

2 tablespoons unsweetened vanilla almond milk

¼ cup pure maple syrup

2 teaspoons pure vanilla extract

Place all the ingredients in a high-powered blender. Blend on high for 5 minutes, until smooth. As the blender mixture warms, the cashews will thicken it. Let the frosting cool for 5 minutes; it will continue to thicken. Then use to ice the cake.

strawberry *milkshake*

3/4 cup unsweetened Homemade Almond Milk (page 223) or store-bought

1 cup frozen strawberries

1/2 teaspoon pure vanilla extract

2 teaspoons agave nectar or organic raw honey

serves 1 • **What girl doesn't like chocolate? My daughter, that's who. This is Avey's special strawberry milkshake. It's simple, delicious, and a great treat to have on a movie night with popcorn!**

Place all the ingredients in a high-powered blender and blend on high until smooth. Pour into a glass and serve.

---

chocolate peanut butter *milkshake*

1/2 cup unsweetened vanilla almond milk

2 tablespoons PBfit Organic Peanut Butter Powder or organic peanut butter

1/2 tablespoon cacao powder

1/2 tablespoon dairy-free chocolate chips

1 frozen banana

Handful of baby spinach (optional)

1 cup ice cubes

serves 1 • **This shake is where it's at. I don't think I can stress this enough: stop what you are doing and make this right now! If you miss ice cream, chocolate, or peanut butter cups, this will hit the spot.**

Place all the ingredients in a high-powered blender and blend on high until smooth. Pour into a glass and serve.

peaches and cream ice cream

1 (15-ounce) can full-fat coconut milk

2½ cups sliced frozen peaches

2 tablespoons agave nectar, pure maple syrup, or organic raw honey

1 teaspoon pure vanilla extract

½ cup Homemade Almond Milk (page 223) (optional)

serves 6 to 8 • **Healthy ice cream! You can add spinach to any of these recipes for a little green punch or serve them as is. The fruit creates beautiful colors in this "nice" cream. Be sure to read the Tip for methods of freezing the ice cream.**

Place all the ingredients, except the almond milk (if using), in a high-powered blender and blend until smooth. Transfer to a freezer container and freeze for at least 3 hours or overnight. When ready to serve, stir in and blend the almond milk for a "scoopable" ice cream (see Tip).

tip: You can also freeze the ice cream in individual servings by using silicone muffin liners. When freezing in a single piece, line the container with parchment. When you remove the container from the freezer, cut the frozen ice cream into chunks that easily fit into your blender. Then add the almond milk and re-blend for perfect scooping consistency.

variations

Vanilla: Omit the peaches.

Strawberry Banana: Substitute 2½ cups frozen strawberries and 1 frozen banana for the frozen peaches.

Tropical Sunshine: Substitute 1 peeled orange, 1 frozen banana, and 1 cup frozen pineapple for the peaches, then add the juice from 1 fresh lime and top with a mint sprig.

dairy-free fudge pops

1/3 cup unsweetened almond milk

1 small ripe avocado, peeled and pitted

2 tablespoons pure maple syrup

1/2 teaspoon pure vanilla extract

2 tablespoons cacao powder

2 tablespoons dairy-free chocolate chips

makes 4 small fudge pops • Who doesn't love a fudgey ice pop? Using avocado is a great way to get healthy fats without sacrificing the creaminess that dairy traditionally brings to this treat. You can also serve this as a chocolate pudding if you forgo the ice step. YUM!

Place all the ingredients in a high-powered blender and blend until smooth and creamy. Freeze in 3-ounce ice pop molds for 4 hours or overnight.

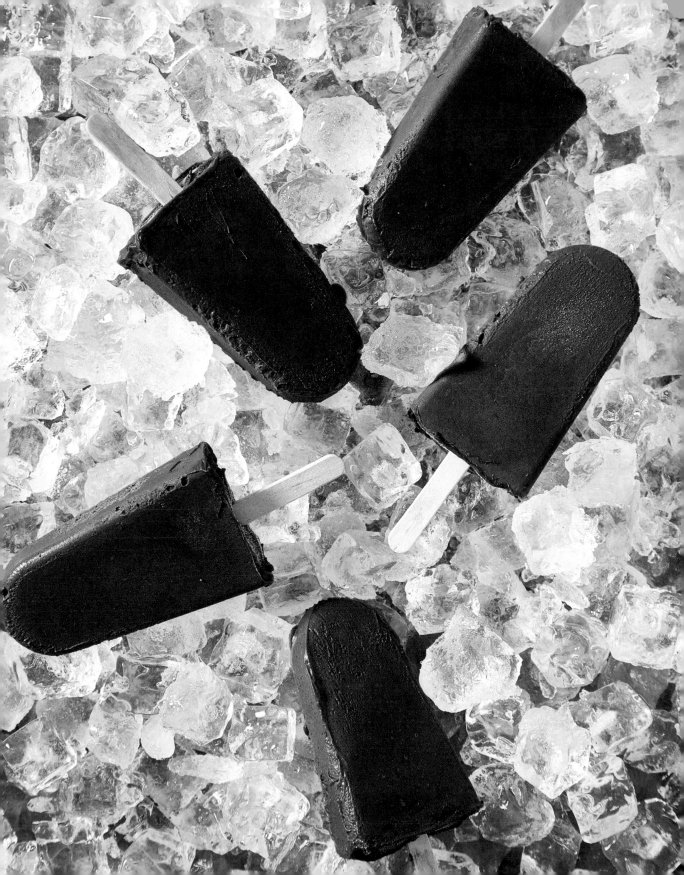

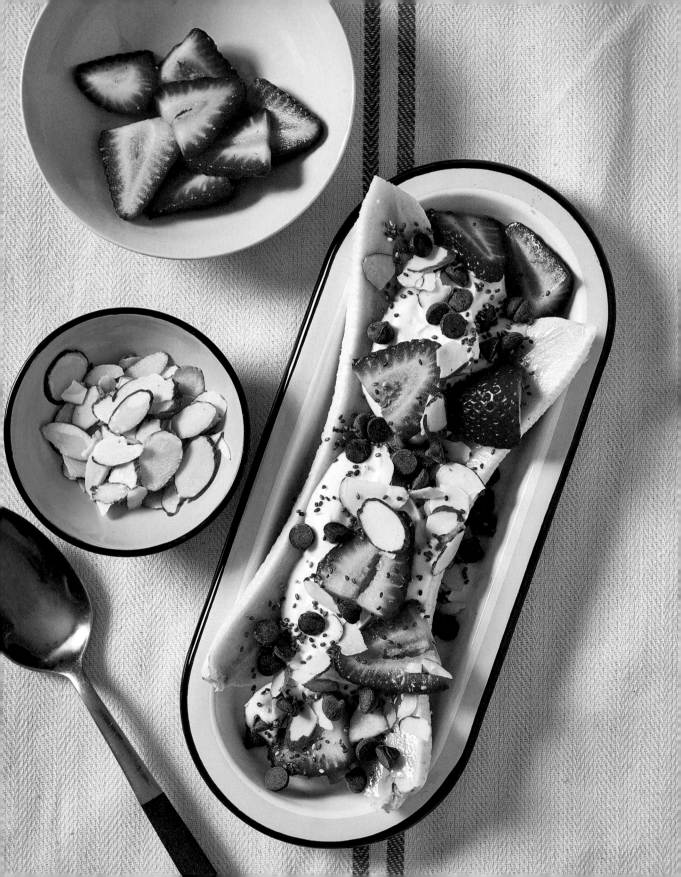

banana split

1 ripe banana, split in half lengthwise

2 tablespoons Coconut Whipped Cream (page 43)

1 tablespoon sliced almonds

1 teaspoon chia seeds

¼ cup sliced strawberries

serves 1 • Here's a healthy take on a classic. Banana Split Night is always a fun time in our house. The sky is the limit here, too. We set up a little sundae bar and let the kids create their own treats. Cherries, granola, chocolate chips, cacao powder—there are limitless variations possible. The recipe serves 1 but the quantities are easily multiplied for the family.

Place the banana in a long narrow dish and top with all the condiments.

skinny margarita

1/3 cup fresh lime juice

1/8 cup Triple Sec

1/4 cup (2 ounces) tequila

2 cups ice cubes

2 tablespoons organic agave nectar

serves 2 • **I love a good margarita. Most diets call for abstaining from alcohol, but I knew that wasn't a realistic lifestyle change for me. Instead, I threw out the sugar-filled mixes and began mixing my own drinks. If you want to feel super-healthy, add a handful of spinach to this margarita. Then you can call it a green smoothie!**

Place all the ingredients in a high-powered blender. Blend until smooth and and there are no ice pieces. Pour into glasses and serve.

mimosa mocktail

1/2 cup sparkling water

1/2 cup fresh orange juice

serves 1 • **Anytime we gather, alcohol is usually involved. I like to feel included, but don't necessarily want to waste my calories on beverages, so I make a special cocktail with sparkling water. Sometimes I use flavored carbonated water and infuse it with fresh-cut fruit.**

Add the water and juice to a glass, stir, and enjoy.

strawberry limeade slurpie

2 limes, juiced

2 tablespoons agave nectar

6 frozen strawberries

1 cup ice cubes

1 teaspoon pure maple syrup

serves 2 to 4 • **This is a spectacular summertime treat—so refreshing on a hot day. You can also use this recipe to make ice pops.**

Place all the ingredients in a high-powered blender and blend until smooth. Pour into glasses and serve immediately.

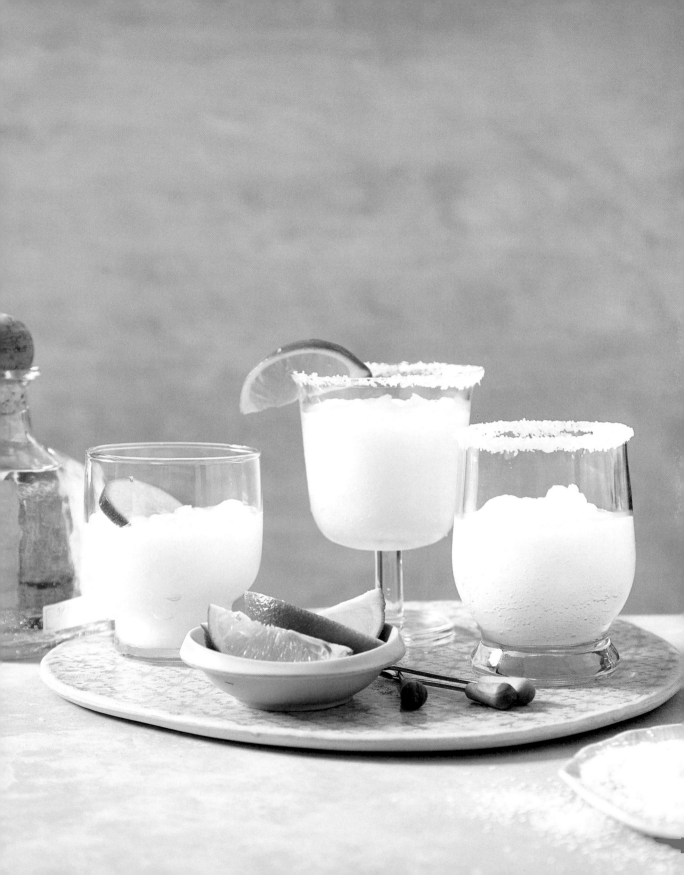

the
BASICS

grain-free
pizza crust

2/3 cup cassava flour, or more
    as needed

1/3 cup arrowroot powder

1 teaspoon sea salt

1/2 teaspoon onion powder

1/2 teaspoon garlic powder

1 egg

2 1/2 tablespoons extra-virgin olive oil

1/3 cup water

Coconut flour, for rolling

One 10-inch crust • Cauliflower pizza crust is all the rage, but for some reason we just can't get into it. So while this recipe isn't necessarily lower in calories than traditional dough, cassava flour doesn't have the same inflammatory side effects as regular flour. This version hits the spot like no other grain-free pizza crust we've tried.

1. Combine the flour, arrowroot, salt, and onion and garlic powders in a medium bowl. Add the egg, oil, and water, then mix well until the mixture forms a ball. Allow the dough to rest for 5 minutes. The ball should not be sticky. If it's sticky, add a little more cassava flour.

2. Sprinkle a sheet of parchment with coconut flour. Flatten the dough with your hands and use a rolling pin to roll out gently into a 10-inch circle. These flours contain no gluten and are not stretchy in nature, so working with the dough will be different from working with wheat flour.

note: To make the pizza, preheat the oven to 425°F. Top the crust with your favorite pizza toppings and use the parchment to slide the pizza onto a baking sheet or pizza stone and bake for 11 minutes. If using a baking sheet, extend the cook time by 2 minutes or until the edges begin to turn golden. The crust comes out better on a preheated pizza stone.

strawberry syrup

1 cup fresh or frozen strawberries

¼ cup pure maple syrup

makes 1 cup • We drizzle this syrup on pancakes, waffles, ice cream, and so much more. Feel free to play around and substitute any fruit you like. Also, here's a neat trick if you have a high-powered blender like a Vitamix: If you mix the ingredients in the blender and then let the mixture stand for 10 minutes, the syrup actually takes on the consistency of a jam that you can use as a spread. If you want to make this even lower in calories, use water and a pinch of stevia instead of the maple syrup.

Place all the ingredients in a blender and blend until smooth.

homemade bone broth

3 pounds meaty bones of choice
   (from chicken parts, beef, lamb,
   pork, or nonoily fish)

4 cups vegetables of choice
   (½ onion, a few carrots, a few
   celery stalks, etc.)

1 tablespoon fresh herbs of choice
   (parsley, basil, etc.)

1 tablespoon apple cider vinegar

1 teaspoon sea salt

makes 3 to 4 quarts • There are so many benefits to making your own broth, whether it be from poultry or meat bones or strictly from vegetables. When we started doing the AIP diet, we began drinking bone broth because it's allergy free and not inflammatory. We like to live a zero waste/low cost lifestyle and making your own broth accomplishes both of those. Note: If you're using beef bones, roast them in the oven at 350°F for 30 minutes before beginning.

1. Place all the ingredients in a pressure cooker and add enough water to fill two-thirds full.

2. Place the lid on the cooker and make sure the pressure knob is in the SEALING position. Using the display panel, select the MANUAL/PRESSURE COOK function, high pressure, and use the +/- buttons until the display reads 90 minutes.

3. When the cooker beeps to let you know it's finished, let it naturally come down from pressure, about 20 minutes.

4. Open the lid of the cooker and strain the broth. Discard the bones and the vegetables. When the broth is completely cool, pour it into jars and store in the refrigerator for up to 10 days.

vegetable broth

4 cups vegetable scraps
(carrots, onions, celery,
bell pepper tops, beet tops,
sweet potato ends, etc.)

5 garlic cloves, crushed

1 dried bay leaf

1 tablespoon minced fresh parsley

1 teaspoon dried rosemary

1 teaspoon dried thyme

$\frac{1}{2}$ teaspoon sea salt

$\frac{1}{4}$ teaspoon black pepper

1 tablespoon extra-virgin olive oil

makes 3 to 4 quarts • **I use vegetable cuttings that I'd normally throw away to make my vegetable stock: the ends of carrots, celery, onions, tomatoes, bell pepper tops, etc. We store all the scraps in gallon freezer bags in the freezer, and once a week I toss them into my pressure cooker with some water. And since we're always looking for ways to help the environment, after we make the vegetable broth, we use the spent vegetables for compost! Keep in mind, though, that there are a few vegetables that don't taste as great in stocks, including leafy greens, broccoli, and cauliflower.**

1. Place all the ingredients in a pressure cooker and add enough water to fill to two-thirds.

2. Place the lid on the cooker and make sure the pressure knob is in the SEALING position. Using the display panel, select the MANUAL/ PRESSURE COOK function, high pressure, and use the +/- buttons until the display reads 40 minutes.

3. When the cooker beeps to let you know it's finished, let it naturally come down from pressure, about 20 minutes.

4. Open the lid of the cooker and strain the broth. Discard the vegetable scraps and the bay leaf. When the broth has cooled completely, pour it into jars and store in the refrigerator for up to 10 days.

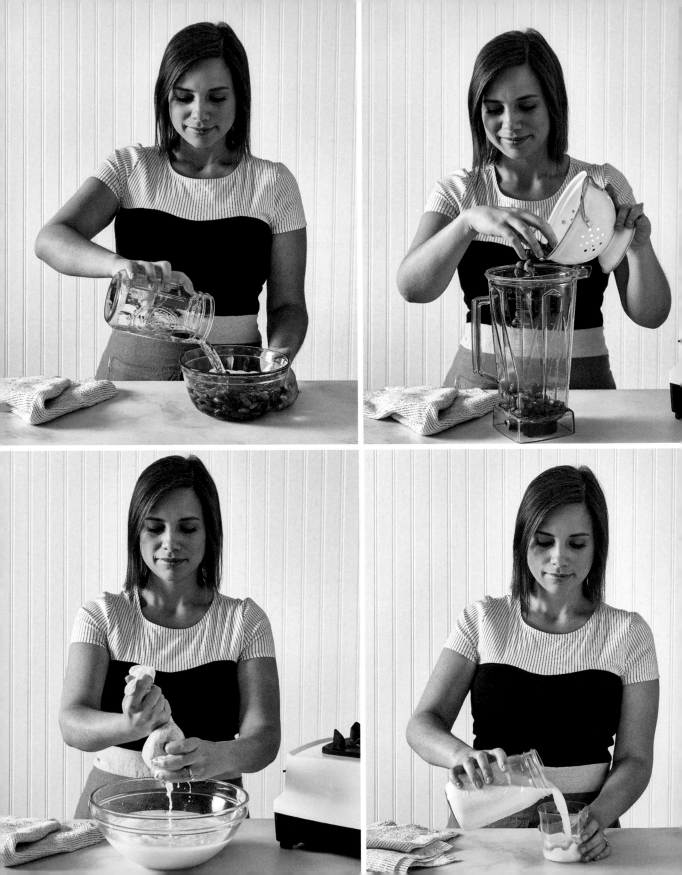

homemade almond milk

1 cup raw almonds

6 cups water

makes 1½ quarts • When I started making healthy choices, I couldn't re-create every meal at once. It was a gradual process. Once I mastered one thing, I went on to the next. Store-bought almond milk isn't actually too expensive, but it was reading the list of ingredients one day that had me thinking I needed to make my own. Once I did, I realized just how easy it was. Almonds are expensive, so don't throw away the pulp; use them for my Almond Pulp Pancakes (page 55).

1. Soak the almonds in 2 cups of the water for 8 hours or overnight. Rinse and drain the almonds.

2. Add the almonds to a high-powered blender along with the remaining 4 cups water. Blend on high until there are no remaining chunks of almonds.

3. Strain the almond milk through a nut milk bag or a piece of cheesecloth, ringing well. Store the almond milk in a glass container in the refrigerator and use within 5 to 7 days. Almond pulp goes rancid quickly so freeze for future use if keeping longer than 2 days.

tip: The almond pulp can also be dehydrated in an oven set to 115°F for 4 to 8 hours.

variation

Vanilla Almond Milk: Add 4 dates and 2 teaspoons pure vanilla extract to the mix when blending.

homemade mayonnaise

1 cup avocado oil, sunflower oil, grapeseed oil, or light olive oil

1 egg, at room temperature

½ teaspoon dried minced onion

½ teaspoon sea salt

Juice of ½ lemon, or 1 teaspoon apple cider vinegar

makes 2 cups • **Ever wonder why store-bought mayonnaise lasts months in the fridge and your homemade version only keeps for seven days? Preservatives! Go preservative free and know exactly what you're putting in your body. We go through a lot of mayo in our house (tuna fish, egg salad, dressings) so we have no trouble using it all up. If you want to make a little less mayo, just use less oil (to make 1 cup of mayo, use ½ cup oil; for ½ cup of mayo, use ¼ cup oil). And if you can't wait for your egg to come to room temperature, you can run it under warm water.**

Place ¼ cup of the oil, the egg, onion, and salt in a wide-mouth mason jar. Use an immersion blender to blend while slowly adding the remaining ¾ cup oil. The slower the drizzle, the thicker the mayonnaise. Once it has emulsified, gently stir in the lemon juice with a spoon. Store in the refrigerator for up to 1 week.

homemade ketchup

1 cup organic tomato sauce

2 tablespoons organic raw honey

1 teaspoon liquid smoke

1 tablespoon organic tomato paste

2 tablespoons red wine vinegar

1 teaspoon dried minced onion

1/2 teaspoon sea salt

makes 1 cup • In the last 100 years, Americans have gone from eating 20 teaspoons of sugar a year to 150 pounds of sugar annually. With the rise of fatty liver disease, it's essential that we pay attention to the food labels on things we purchase. This is especially true for the foods we give to our children—childhood obesity and Type 2 diabetes are at all-time highs among our little ones. There are small but mighty changes you can make at home, including this ketchup. If you're not up to making your own, however, there are several brands that have reduced sodium and sugar, made with whole-food ingredients. Just stay away from anything that contains high-fructose corn syrup!

Place all the ingredients in a wide-mouth mason jar and blend with an immersion blender until combined. Store in the refrigerator for up to 2 weeks.

pressure cooker *black beans*

1 (16-ounce) package
   dried black beans

makes 3 pounds • **As a base for several of my go-to recipes, I like to make a big batch of these and freeze what I don't use for future use.**

1. Cover the beans with water and soak for 4 hours or overnight. Rinse and drain.

2. Place the beans in the pressure cooker and barely cover with water.

3. Place the lid on the cooker and make sure the pressure knob is in the SEALING position. Using the display panel, select the MANUAL/ PRESSURE COOK function, high pressure, and use the +/- buttons until the display reads 12 minutes.

4. When the cooker beeps to let you know it's finished, let it naturally come down from pressure until the display reads LO:35.

5. Open the lid and spoon out to use.

pressure cooker *chickpeas*

1 (16-ounce) package
dried chickpeas

makes 3 pounds • **A good source of protein, these are used in several of my go-to recipes.**

1. In a large bowl, cover the chickpeas with water and soak for 8 hours or overnight. Make sure to cover the beans with more water than you think they will need when hydrating. They'll absorb quite a bit.

2. Drain and rinse the chickpeas and add to a pressure cooker. Barely cover the beans with water; it's okay if you see a few beans peeking out through the surface of the water.

3. Place the lid on the cooker and make sure the pressure knob is in the SEALING position. Using the display panel, select the MANUAL/ PRESSURE COOK function, high pressure, and use the +/- buttons until the display reads 25 minutes.

4. When the cooker beeps to let you know it's finished, let it naturally come down from pressure until the display reads LO:3. Switch the pressure knob from the SEALING to the VENTING position.

5. Open the lid. You will notice that the chickpeas are covered in a white weblike substance; don't be alarmed. Just rinse and drain them. They are ready to go in whatever recipe you'd like to use them in. They're good for about 5 days in the refrigerator or they last for months in the freezer.

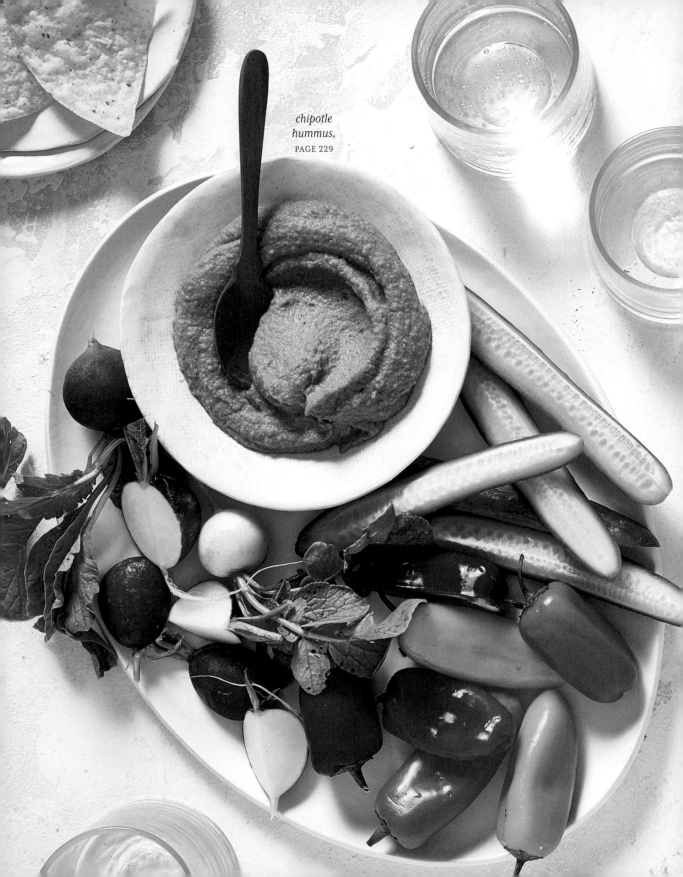

chipotle hummus, PAGE 229

chipotle hummus

1 cup cooked chickpeas, homemade (page 227) or canned, rinsed and drained

½ cup avocado oil

1 tablespoon tahini (optional)

1 chipotle pepper in adobo sauce, or 2 if you like it spicy!

½ teaspoon sea salt

½ teaspoon ground cumin

1 teaspoon minced garlic

4 teaspoons fresh lemon juice

makes 2 cups • **This is the best hummus ever. I was never really a fan of hummus—until I began making my own. Now it's something I always keep on hand, along with crisp cucumbers, for snacking. I love to serve this dynamite hummus at parties, too. I always get asked for the recipe. It's so good!**

Place all the ingredients in a food processor or a blender and blend on high until smooth and creamy. Serve with tortilla chips or fresh raw veggies.

veggie dip,
PAGE 230

cilantro jalapeño hummus,
PAGE 230

veggie *dip*

1 cup mashed ripe avocado

½ tablespoon fresh lime juice

½ teaspoon garlic powder

¼ teaspoon sea salt

makes 1 cup • **Here's a veggie dip made with avocado—you can't get healthier than that! My kids love to build their own lunch trays. I lay out lots of raw veggies and some healthy deli meats, and they build their own plates using this dip as the dressing.**

Place all the ingredients in a bowl and stir to combine. Serve with raw veggies. Consume within 48 hours.

cilantro jalapeño *hummus*

1 cup cooked chickpeas, homemade (page 227), or store-bought, rinsed and drained

½ cup avocado oil

1 tablespoon tahini (optional)

½ cup fresh cilantro, including stems, chopped

¼ cup diced jalapeño (ribs and seeds removed for less spice)

1 teaspoon ground cumin

1 teaspoon dried minced onion

½ teaspoon sea salt

makes 2 cups • **This hummus is incredible! It's great served with raw veggies or tortilla chips, but even better on a tostada or in a taco. This is a perfect dip to bring to a potluck party as well.**

Place all the ingredients in a food processor or a blender and blend on high until smooth and creamy. Serve with tortilla chips or fresh raw veggies. Store in the refrigerator for up to a week.

taco *seasoning*

1½ tablespoons chili powder

2 teaspoons dried minced onion

1 teaspoon garlic powder

1 teaspoon ground cumin

1 teaspoon sea salt

½ teaspoon cayenne

½ teaspoon smoked paprika

makes ¼ cup • **Store-bought taco seasonings are full of things like "natural flavors," which could be a hidden term for MSG and other preservatives. If you're able, it is best to make your own taco seasoning. I developed this recipe with McCormicks Traditional Taco Seasoning in mind, and it won't disappoint!**

Combine all the ingredients in a mason jar and seal. The taco seasoning will keep for up to 6 months.

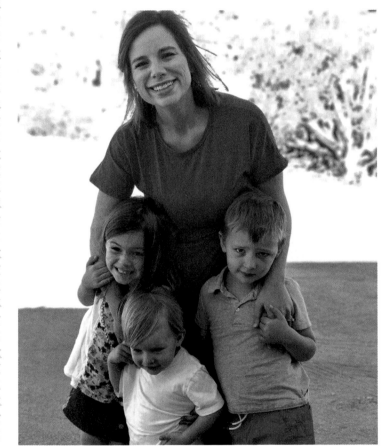

ACKNOWLEDGMENTS

Brady, God only knows where I'd be without you. You introduced me to romaine lettuce, the Vitamix, and the Instant Pot®! Clearly, you're a brilliant human being. You made me a wife, a mom, and a better person. I couldn't have done any of this without you. Thank you for loving me when I didn't love myself very much. You're truly my better half and the love of my life. This book is because of you.

Avey, Ben, and Noah, thank you for being my brave first testers, my best encouragers, dubbing me "Greatest Cooker Ever," and for sharing me so that I can share my passions with others. You are the reason I stopped making excuses and changed my life. The depth of my love for you knows no bounds.

Mom and Dad, thank you for all the free babysitting, free therapy, and believing that I could do anything. You make me believe it, too.

Aunt Kim, my love of cooking was born out of my love for you.

Grandma, some of my earliest memories in the kitchen are of you making wonderful treats. Many of these recipes have your influence behind them. Thank you.

Grandma Sharon, not many people would drop everything on a dime and drive 4,000 miles roundtrip just because their granddaughter needed help with a cookbook. Your presence in my life is a treasure.

Andy Barzvi, thank you for seeing me and roping me into this adventure with your big charismatic personality. Amazing agent and fabulous friend.

Donna Loffredo and the Harmony team, well, none of this would have happened without ya'll! Literally. Thank you for taking a chance on my dream and bringing it to life.

Diana Baroni, for taking a chance on this little project of mine and seeing the promise before anyone else. Thank you.

Tammy Blake, for all the behind-the-scenes calls, emails, and going to bat for me and Instant Loss. It's been a pleasure working with you.

Helene Dujardin, your genius breathed life into the words on the pages. Thank you for welcoming us into your home and your creative spaces. Your photos reflect your character, impeccably beautiful and dignified.

Tami Hardeman, it was day two of the photoshoot when I realized that there's not a single food that exists on this planet that you can't make look pretty. (Four potatoes, lol!) Thank you for your patience, your care, and your extraordinary talent. This book is so much better for having you.

Lisa Rovick, for the lunches, belly laughs, and testing the brownies four different times. It was an absolute pleasure to work beside you for eight days as we knocked out the photography. Thank you for all of your honesty and your feedback. Your insight was invaluable.

Mindi Shapiro, you quite possibly have more dishes than anyone I've ever known, and girl, can you work those dishes! Thank you for all the beautiful treasures you lent to the photos in this book and for your artistic abilities to see a masterpiece and construct the bones so that the rest can be painted.

Instant Loss community, all of this is for you and because of you! Instant Loss would have never been born without you! All I wanted to do was encourage one person who needed help, like me, and you gave me a platform to reach millions. This is our story. Every life that is touched and changed is a collective effort that you had a hand in. I owe all this to you!

Jesus, savior, redeemer, king, and friend. I owe all that I have to you.

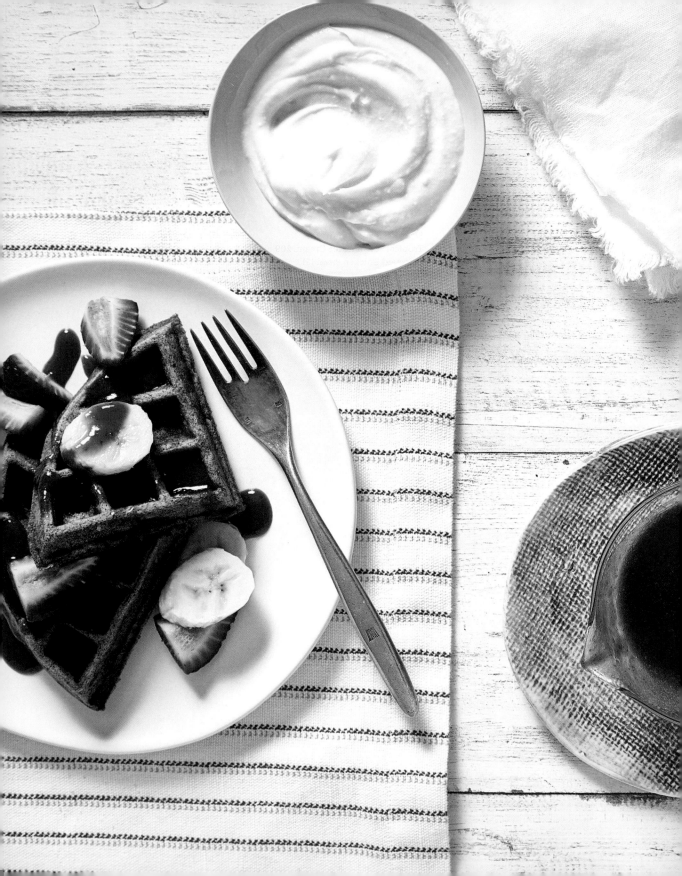

INDEX

ABOUT THE AUTHOR

Brittany Williams, a mother of three, a blogger, and a self-proclaimed lover of food, decided to make a big change in her diet by removing processed snacks, take-out, and high-calorie meals from her family's menus. And she replaced those foods with healthier meals she could make in her Instant Pot. She has since lost 125 pounds and has been featured in media, including *Good Morning America, Today,* and more. Find her online at InstantLoss.com or instagram.com/instantloss.

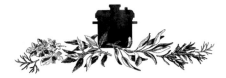